You've Hit Menopause: Now What?

3 Simple Steps to Restoring Hormone Balance

George Gillson MD, PhD
Tracy Marsden BScPharm

The information in this book is not meant to be a substitute for the advice of a competent health professional. We strongly urge you to discuss what you learn from this book with your health care provider.

ISBN 0-9732962-1-6

Printed in Canada
Second Edition, October 2004

Printed by Blitzprint, Calgary AB

Rocky Mountain Analytical Corp.
Unit A, 253147 Bearspaw Road NW
Calgary, Alberta T3L 2P5
Copyright October, 2004

Website: www.rmalab.com
Email: info@rmalab.com

ACKNOWLEDGEMENTS

The authors wish to thank the following people for their assistance in preparing and reviewing the manuscript of the first and second editions:

Candace Burch, Melanie Faulknor, Bob Geldreich, Bob Heim, Sue Horton, Maureen Kitchur, Serena Kolodka, Bill and Sally Marsden, Jim Paoletti, Vivian Pritchard, Jeanette Queen, Ellen San Augustin, Todd Spetter, Larry Thorne, Nadine Velasco, and Dr. David Zava

A big thank you to Linda Sharp of North Vancouver, BC for her designing genius.

We would also like to thank Holly Roy and Aaron Murzyn of Pumpkin Innovation in Edmonton for their Public Relations support and expertise.

We are indebted to Alexis Gillson, Dan Motyka, Faralee Chanin, and Darrell and Alison Jones for their support in getting this project off the ground

ABOUT THE AUTHORS

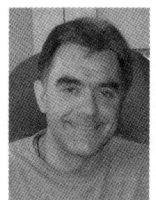 **Dr. George Gillson** is the President and Medical Director of Rocky Mountain Analytical, a laboratory specializing in salivary hormone analysis. Dr. Gillson received a PhD in chemistry from the University of Alberta before earning his MD from the University of Calgary. He practised Family Medicine for six years before moving to the Tahoma Clinic to work with Jonathan Wright MD, one of the pioneers of the nutritional-biochemical approach to chronic illness and disease prevention. Dr. Gillson also consulted for several laboratories in the area of steroid hormone analysis. Dr. Gillson has experience as a family doctor, understands the role of the laboratory in the practise of medicine, and has solid expertise in the nutritional-natural approach to medicine.

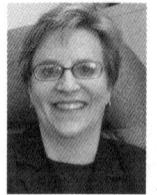 **Tracy Marsden** is Vice-President of Rocky Mountain Analytical. She received a Bachelor of Science degree from the University of Alberta prior to earning her Pharmacy degree. Tracy practised in community pharmacy for fifteen years and did private consultations in natural health for several years. She completed a Diploma in Homeopathic Pharmacy and was awarded a Fellowship in the British Institute of Homeopathy in 1996. Tracy teaches, writes and consults to health professionals, the natural products industry, and pharmacy students on the subject of natural medicines.

TABLE OF CONTENTS

AN INTRODUCTORY HORMONE TALE

Ready, Fire, then Aim

Once upon a time, the pharmaceutical giants Searle, Upjohn and Wyeth-Ayerst hired a fellow named Robert A. Wilson MD to write a book extolling the virtues of estrogen supplementation for women after menopause. The take-home message from Dr. Wilson's book was basically this: if women didn't take estrogen after menopause, they were doomed to become unattractive hags and die prematurely. Women didn't take kindly to the thought that they would shrivel up and die without estrogen, and their physicians didn't want to be responsible for letting that happen either. The net result was that sales of prescription, patented oral estrogen began to climb, and didn't look back. Unfortunately, Dr. Wilson neglected to mention one detail: there really wasn't much research supporting the benefits of oral estrogen, especially estrogens from another species (pregnant mare's urine being the most common source). Pharmaceutical companies led the charge for hormone replacement in the 1960's and physicians willingly followed: a classic case of Ready, Fire – *then* Aim.

After a few years of giving women fairly high oral doses of non-human estrogens, we discovered that this approach led to an increased risk of cancer of the uterine endometrium or lining of the uterus. We had a chance at that point, to step back and reassess what we were doing. We could have added progesterone, the natural hormone produced by the ovaries every month, to oppose the stimulating effect of the horse estrogen. We could have questioned our use of horse estrogen in human beings. We could have questioned the wisdom of *swallowing* hormones, which normally trickle directly into the blood from the ovaries. Instead, we kept the horse estrogen, and added oral medroxyprogesterone acetate (MPA), a synthetic, patentable molecule similar, but not identical; to the body's own progesterone. To be sure, MPA effectively suppressed the development of endometrial cancer, but in retrospect it was probably the worst possible partner for the horse estrogen, as we will discuss.

Time went on and sales continued to grow. Premarin® (conjugated estrogens from pregnant mare's urine) became the number one selling prescription drug in the United States, and hormone replacement therapy (HRT) became a billion dollar industry. In the research world, clouds were appearing on the horizon, but few physicians were watching the weather. Studies were accumulating that showed oral estrogen was likely associated with a small but definite increase in breast cancer, and that addition of MPA to the mix increased the risk. Studies on primates showed that even though estrogens exerted positive effects on the cardiovascular system, MPA opposed those benefits if the two were given together. Studies also showed that MPA given alone as a contraceptive had adverse effects on bone density. The clouds on the horizon were gathering for a storm!

THE WOMEN'S HEALTH INITIATIVE STUDY (WHIS) Key Points

Premarin® and Provera® arm

THE STUDY

- 16,608 postmenopausal women aged 50-79 years with an intact uterus.
- Women received either Premarin® 0.625mg and Provera® 2.5mg daily (8506 women) *or* placebo (8102 women).
- Outcomes measured included heart disease, invasive breast cancer, colorectal cancer, hip fracture, endometrial cancer, stroke and blood clots in lungs
- A global index summarizing the balance of risks versus benefits was also used.

RESULTS

- The study was stopped early because the global index indicated that on balance, the harm from using Premarin® plus Provera® was greater than the benefit.
- Compared to placebo, Premarin® plus Provera® users had:
  - 41% more strokes
  - 29% more heart attacks
  - Twice as many blood clots
  - 26% more breast cancer
  - 37% *less* colorectal cancer
  - 33% *fewer* hip fractures
  - 76% increase in Alzheimer's Dementia

The WHIS proved that oral dosing with non-human and synthetic hormones in the form of Premarin® and Provera® was more harmful to women than giving them a placebo.

By the end of the 1980's numerous studies had been done looking at the effects of hormones in animals, human cells and humans. The papers written on the subject could easily fill a room. Despite mounting evidence of increased breast cancer and cardiovascular risks, there was still enough data to suggest that estrogens *should* be good for the heart and *were* good for the bones, the brain, the urogenital system and the skin. No one was too worried.

Eventually, in an attempt to resolve some of the apparent contradictions, various large trials of HRT were launched, studying thousands of women, looking at multiple outcomes to determine whether the benefits outweighed the risks. In the summer of 2002, the storm finally broke. The Women's Health Initiative examined combined HRT in over 16,000 women and found that the risks of combined horse estrogen and MPA outweighed the benefits. An anti-HRT backlash, whose effects will be felt by women for decades, was unleashed.

Therein lies the purpose of this book. The backlash against HRT is causing needless suffering for many women in menopause. Our aim is to clear up the confusion around hormone replacement, offer 3 simple strategies to determine whether a woman would benefit from hormone replacement *and* look at the best options for HRT in light of recent research findings. We are ready: we have a clear target: let's fire away!

CHAPTER ONE

Hormone Help or Hormone Heartache?

The big hormone news of 2002 was that the hormone *help* women were promised turned out to be hormone *heartache* for some. For decades, women were told that hormone replacement would keep them young and healthy. Now women are being warned that some forms of hormone replacement can actually *increase* their risk of heart disease and breast cancer. The early closure of the combined conjugated estrogens and synthetic progestin arm of the Women's Health Initiative Study (see inset page iii) caused many women to rush to their physicians and demand to be taken off hormone replacement therapy (HRT). Physicians whose knowledge of hormones was limited to *off-the-shelf* products, had no alternatives to offer. In fact, many physicians were caught off guard by the results of this study. Instead of demonstrating an overall benefit for this form of hormone replacement, the WHIS showed an *increase* in heart disease, breast cancer, stroke and blood clots in the women taking Premarin® and Provera®. This caused many women and their physicians to abandon hormone replacement completely, with unfortunate consequences for some.

1

The following two cases are typical of how the results of the WHIS have impacted the lives of menopausal women:

Jane

Jane is a post-menopausal woman who had a complete hysterectomy (removal of the ovaries and uterus) ten years ago, and was then put on an estrogen skin patch. She was told that because her uterus had been removed, she didn't need progesterone. Jane stopped her patch after the results of the WHIS were made public. She's afraid that using the patch will increase her risk of heart disease and breast cancer. And now, she complains: "I'm suffering severe vaginal dryness; I'm having trouble sleeping; I'm depressed and I just don't feel like myself anymore." Jane believes the risks of HRT outweigh the benefits, but now she is experiencing all the symptoms of a hormone deficiency. Is Jane at risk by continuing to use an estrogen patch? Probably not. Jane's patch contains an estrogen called estradiol, which is identical to what the body produces naturally. Delivering hormone through the skin (transdermally) is better than giving hormones orally because transdermal delivery is more efficient and is closer to the way hormones are distributed naturally in the body. Jane has no family history of breast cancer, and she is using a very low dose of estrogen. Continued use of the estradiol patch, and regular monitoring of estradiol and other hormone levels is probably a good long-term strategy for Jane. However, Jane should consider using *bio-identical* progesterone to balance her estradiol, as her body did on its own before her ovaries were removed. Progesterone helps the body make better use of estrogens, and prevents symptoms of estrogen excess. There is also evidence that progesterone may help reduce the risk of breast cancer and that it's good for the heart and blood vessels. Jane has experienced needless distress by stopping her hormone patch.

Trudy

Trudy has been using Premarin® and Provera® for 5 years, ever since she hit menopause. She still has her ovaries and uterus, and she has a family history of heart disease. Trudy says: "I don't care what the study says. I'm not stopping my hormones. I suffered a long time with hot flashes and sleep problems before my doctor finally put me on hormones. I'm not going back!" Trudy doesn't have to give up hormone therapy, but she needs to change her hormone regimen. The synthetic progestin MPA is known to increase the overall risk of heart disease in postmenopausal women. Trudy's physician doesn't really want to keep her on Premarin® but doesn't know what else to suggest. Trudy would be better off using natural progesterone, identical to what is produced in the body, instead of MPA, especially given her family history of heart disease. Trudy would also be well served by using a transdermal form of estradiol, rather than oral conjugated estrogens. Hormone delivered through the skin is similar to natural production of estrogen by the ovaries, and has a lower risk of causing blood clots than the oral form.

There are many other women out there with *undiagnosed* problems. They have multiple symptoms that may be related to hormone deficiencies and imbalances, and although they *suspect* hormone involvement, they don't know for sure whether or not their problems are hormone related. Physicians rarely test women's hormone levels, and even if they had laboratory evidence of deficiencies, they would probably still hesitate to prescribe hormones. Why is that? Physicians are conflicted: they are torn between the drug company literature that says: "Premarin® and Provera® help women" and what the research shows: "the risk of breast cancer and heart disease increases significantly in women taking conjugated estrogens and MPA". This conflict has resulted in a kind of prescribing paralysis for physicians; they're afraid to prescribe *any* hormones, even when there is a clearly demonstrated deficiency! Physicians are also reluctant to go outside the guidelines set by various expert panels for fear that they will be accused of not following the standard of practice. Family doctors receive very little education on hormones, and most don't have the time to evolve their own strategies based on their readings of the scientific literature. So for a variety of reasons, thousands of women have been left without good information on their hormone options, and are now desperately seeking solutions to their problems

The good news is that hormone help *can* come from using the right hormones at the right dose and delivering them in the right way. This is called bio-identical hormone replacement, or BHRT (see page 5). Unfortunately, physicians don't get a lot of information about hormone therapies in general, and even less about bio-identical or natural hormones. For example, there are an embarrassing number of physicians, researchers and pharmacists who still don't understand that the synthetic progestin MPA (medroxyprogesterone acetate) is *not* progesterone. Many health professionals use the term progesterone to describe MPA, which is a *synthetic* progestin. Studies have consistently shown that synthetic progestins do not have the same effects as progesterone, and this will be discussed in some detail later. Dr. John Lee did women a great service by bringing research on progesterone into the public eye (read *What Your Doctor May Not Tell You About Pre-Menopause)*. And, more recently, Suzanne Somers' book *The Sexy Years* has increased awareness of BHRT as a practical alternative to conventional HRT. We will discuss some specifics of Ms. Somers' book in Chapter Four.

BIO-IDENTICAL HORMONE REPLACEMENT (BHRT)

BHRT refers to the therapeutic use of hormones that are identical in every way to the hormones produced naturally in the body. Bio-identical hormones used in BHRT include estradiol, estrone, estriol, progesterone and testosterone. DHEA and androstenedione are also bio-identical hormones, but are not available in Canada. Cortisol may be supplemented in cases of cortisol deficiency, but cortisol replacement is not normally considered part of BHRT.

There is no reason why any woman in menopause should have to suffer. There are alternatives! Properly balanced hormones can relieve unpleasant symptoms and may even help prevent disease. In many cases, lifestyle and nutritional strategies are sufficient to alleviate many menopause symptoms. But, for some women, lifestyle and dietary changes aren't enough to stem the tide of menopausal symptoms. Women and their physicians must be educated regarding the benefits of bio-identical hormone replacement.

We want to help clear up the confusion surrounding hormone replacement, and look at how bio-identical hormone replacement can help relieve symptoms, likely *without* the long-term risks associated with other HRT approaches. Using the right kind of hormones, in the right way and at the right dose can improve health and relieve distressing symptoms. It's time to learn from the mistakes of the past and move forward with new hormone replacement strategies.

We have developed a simple 3-Step plan to help women and their physicians decide whether hormone replacement is necessary, and to determine the best options for replacing hormones. Although the need for hormone replacement is by no means universal, countless women have obtained benefit from the judicious use of hormones. Hormones are not the enemy; the enemy is ignorance.

CHAPTER TWO

Hormone Basics

Before taking aim to resolve hormone replacement issues, it's important to have a thorough understanding of what hormones do. In simplest terms, hormones are chemical messengers that travel through blood, enter tissues and regulate cell function. Hormones may influence cell activity without involving hormone receptors, but we are mostly concerned with the *direct* effects of hormones, which result from interaction with specific receptors. Hormones act on receptors the way a key fits into a lock (see Figure 1). Putting the hormone *key* in the receptor *lock* helps to regulate functions controlled by that hormone. If the key is slightly different (i.e. a non-identical synthetic hormone), it might fit the lock, but not open the same doors as the proper key (natural hormone). Synthetic hormones may also leave the door open too long, or slam it shut too soon. Hormones interact frequently both with receptor sites and with one another, and each hormone can act in many different ways. There are dozens of hormones in the human body and it often takes several hormones to get a specific response. For example, four hormones are needed to stimulate the release of an egg at ovulation. Because hormones are extremely interdependent and their interactions so complex, it is

7

essential to maintain the proper balance of hormones and use the right keys for the hormone receptor locks (bio-identical hormones).

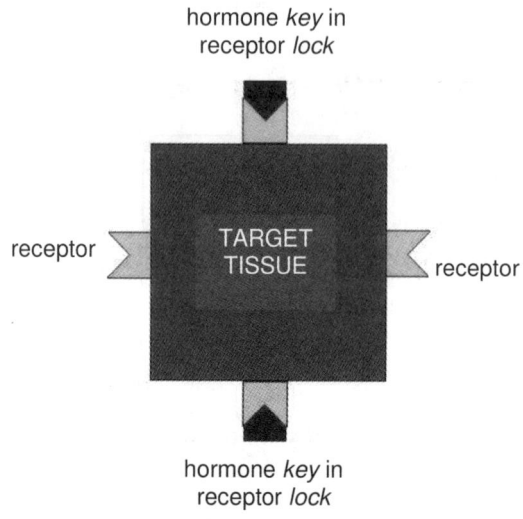

Figure 1

WHERE ARE HORMONES MADE?

Estrogens, androgens, progesterone, and cortisol are all part of the group of hormones known as steroid hormones. Steroid hormones are manufactured in the body from cholesterol, the chemical backbone of all the steroid hormones. Most people don't realize that men and women share all the same hormones. The relative amounts of each hormone obviously differ, but the fact is that both sexes require steroid hormones for survival. These hormones fall into one of the following categories: estrogens, androgens, progesterone, or glucocorticoids.

Estrogens are a hormone class, or group of similar hormone molecules. The estrogens are commonly thought of as exclusively female hormones, but are also essential for men. Conversely, the androgens and their precursors (the molecules that androgens are made from) are often considered male hormones, but are also essential to women. The most common androgen is testosterone. Dehydroepiandrosterone (DHEA) and androstenedione are both androgen precursors. Progesterone is the lone hormone in its class, although it can serve as a precursor for cortisol. Cortisol is one of the primary hormones of the glucocorticoid family.

In women, sex steroid hormones are produced primarily by the ovaries and adrenal glands. Hormones produced by the ovaries are depicted in Figure 2.

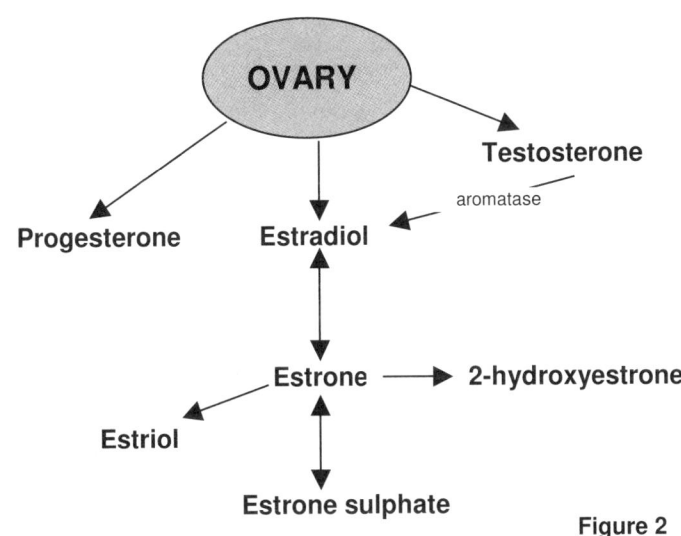

Figure 2

The adrenal glands are small glands located on top of the kidneys. The adrenal glands release the stress hormones adrenaline and cortisol, as well as the androgen precursor, DHEA. Androstenedione is formed from DHEA, and is a building block for both testosterone and the estrogens. Figure 3 shows a simplified diagram of the production of hormones via the adrenal glands.

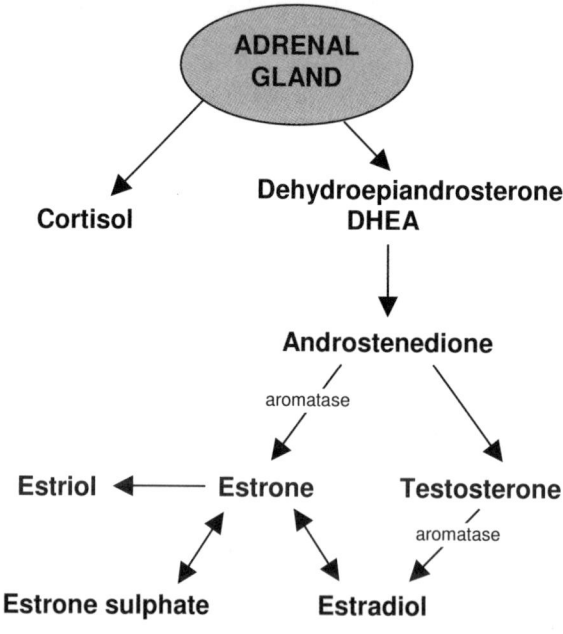

Figure 3

The conversion of each hormone to another in the pathway requires specific enzymes, which in turn require specific vitamins and minerals. Consequently, vitamin and mineral deficiencies can have a significant effect on hormone balance. Hormone production is also affected by other factors. Aromatase, a very important enzyme found in fat cells, converts androgens to estrogens. Women who are overweight have more aromatase and therefore convert more androstenedione to estrone. As a result, obese women often experience few estrogen deficiency symptoms. Conversely, thin women are more prone to estrogen deficiency symptoms.

The Critical Role of the Adrenal Glands

The importance of the adrenal glands in the production of hormones cannot be over-emphasized. The adrenal glands produce sex hormones throughout the life cycle, but are the *most* important source of sex hormones after menopause.

Pre-Menopause: Prior to menopause, the ovaries are the major producers of estrogens and progesterone. However, almost 40% of pre-menopausal estrogen comes from the adrenal glands. A small amount is secreted directly from the adrenal glands as estradiol or estrone, but most is made from androstenedione via aromatase. About half a woman's testosterone comes from DHEA released by the adrenal glands. Progesterone is also produced by the adrenal glands, but virtually all the progesterone produced in the adrenals is used to make cortisol.

Post-Menopause: Once menopause has been reached, the adrenal glands become the primary source for estrogens and testosterone. The ovaries continue to turn out small amounts of estradiol and testosterone, but the majority comes via conversion from DHEA and androstenedione (see Figure 3). Women who have had a complete hysterectomy (see inset) are similar to postmenopausal women in that they are completely reliant on their adrenal glands for hormone production.

A WOMAN'S GUIDE TO GYNAECOLOGICAL SURGERIES

Hysterectomy refers to the removal of the uterus.

Oophorectomy is the removal of one or both ovaries.

Complete Hysterectomy is the term used to describe the removal of both the ovaries and the uterus. This is also often referred to as surgical menopause.

Post-menopausal women and women who have undergone surgical menopause rely heavily on adrenal hormone production, and any reduction in adrenal function can accelerate the development of hormone deficiencies. Stress, poor diet, lack of sleep, and excessive caffeine consumption all adversely affect the adrenal glands. Stress releases large amounts of cortisol, which causes hormone production to be diverted from the manufacture of DHEA. Chronic high stress may also affect progesterone levels because progesterone is a precursor for cortisol. Nutrition is another important factor. Diets high in simple carbohydrates and refined sugars require extra amounts of the vitamins and minerals the adrenal glands need to do the job of making hormones. Conversely, ensuring an adequate intake of vitamins and minerals can assist adrenal hormone production. Caffeine prolongs the adrenal response to stress, which aggravates adrenal hormone deficiencies. In other words, if you have high cortisol and drink coffee, the effects of cortisol are going to last longer. Continual production of excessive amounts of cortisol leads to adrenal exhaustion. The bottom line is: adrenal exhaustion results in reduced levels of DHEA and androstenedione, the required precursors of estrogens and testosterone!

The body wisely offers multiple means for producing sex hormones, primarily through the ovaries but also by the adrenal glands. Since ovarian production of hormones drops dramatically at menopause, women must look after their adrenal glands. Healthy eating, relaxation and avoidance of caffeine are important steps in achieving and maintaining healthy adrenals. Hormones are essential to life and deficiencies and imbalances can seriously affect a woman's health.

WHAT DO HORMONES DO?

We've established that hormones fit into receptor locks, but where are these locks and what do the androgens, estrogens, progesterone and cortisol do when they get there? We'll look at each group of hormones, discuss their general purpose and look at how they interact. Chapter 3 will look at the specifics of the menstrual cycle and how hormone changes lead to menopause.

Estrogens

Estrogen receptors are found in cells throughout the body, including sites in bone, brain, blood vessels, bladder, breast, thyroid gland and the reproductive organs. Estrogens are responsible for the development of the female secondary sex characteristics such as breast development, and play a critical role in the menstrual cycle.

There are numerous naturally occurring human estrogens, but the most widely recognized are estradiol, estrone and estriol. All the estrogens interact with estrogen receptors, but not necessarily to the same degree. Each estrogen has a different affinity, or *liking* for the estrogen receptor. The stronger the estrogen, the greater its affinity for the receptor and the greater the estrogenic effect it will have.

CONJUGATED ESTROGENS

Estrogens circulate freely in the bloodstream, but also undergo conjugation by the liver. Conjugation is the process by which estrogens are changed into more water-soluble forms by the attachment of sugar molecules and molecules such as sulphate and glutathione. Although conjugated estrogens are usually not considered *active* estrogens, they can in fact be converted back into active forms.

Estradiol

Estradiol is the strongest of the estrogens and is the main estrogen released by the ovaries. Estradiol is also produced via androstenedione from the adrenal glands. Estradiol is the primary estrogen of the menstrual cycle and is responsible for building up the endometrium (lining of the uterus).

Estrone

Estrone is next in strength after estradiol. Estradiol released from the ovaries can be converted into estrone. It is also produced from androstenedione released by the adrenal glands. Estrone is the main post-menopausal estrogen, and can be converted to either estriol or estradiol as needed.

Estrone Sulphate (E1S)

Estrone sulphate is the most abundant estrogen in the body. More than half of all estrogen produced by, or introduced into the body of either sex winds up being stored as estrone sulphate. In fact, estrone sulphate levels for men and post-menopausal women are very comparable. The sulphate form does not act directly on cells, as it cannot fit into the receptor *locks*. It can, however, be converted into estradiol, the most potent estrogen.

2 Hydroxyestrone (2OHE1)

2-hydroxyestrone is not usually considered an active estrogen, but it is a major estrogen breakdown product, and likely has a role in balancing the action of stronger estrogens. Evidence points to a protective role for 2-hydroxyestrone against breast cancer. In fact, progesterone and indole-3-carbinol are compounds widely considered to be protective against breast cancer, and they both enhance the formation of 2-hydroxyestrone.

Many practitioners advocate testing the serum or urine ratio between 2-hydroxyestrone and 16-hydroxyestrone (16OHE1). They believe that a low ratio of 2OHE1 to 16OHE1 is predictive of increased breast cancer risk. This presumes that 16OHE1 is a breast cancer carcinogen; and there is very little solid scientific evidence that this is true. Furthermore, the ratio of 2OHE1 to 16OHE1 changes throughout the menstrual cycle and indeed throughout the life cycle. In fact, high 2OHE1 to 16OHE1 ratio in *pre-*

menopausal women may be weakly associated with a lower incidence of breast cancer, but this same high ratio in *post*-menopausal women is actually associated with an *increased* incidence of breast cancer. In the end, there is no solid evidence that maintenance of a high ratio of 2OHE1 to 16OHE1 will afford protection against breast cancer. Nevertheless, it is likely that having a high level of 2OHE1, irrespective of the 16OHE1 level, will offer some protection against breast cancer.

Estriol

Compared to estradiol and estrone, estriol is the weakest of the three common natural estrogens, but studies indicate it is strong enough to produce estrogenic effects. Estriol is produced from estrone as shown in Figure 2. Estriol levels are very high during pregnancy, and this suggests that estriol is unlikely to be toxic, since the fetus is also exposed to high levels.

Progesterone

The name progesterone refers to its ability to **pro**mote **gest**ation (pregnancy). In fact, progesterone is essential for the maintenance of pregnancy. Progesterone is also the principal hormone of the second half of the menstrual cycle, the luteal phase. Natural progesterone, bio-identical progesterone and progesterone all refer to progesterone produced by the body. Like estrogen receptors, progesterone receptors are found throughout the body: in the brain, bone, breast, bladder, blood vessels, thyroid gland, and reproductive organs. After a hysterectomy, women are often started on estrogen replacement, but are told they don't need progesterone because they no longer have a uterus! This is completely wrong. *All* the body's tissues need exposure to both hormones for optimum health.

Progesterone is produced naturally in the ovaries, and in small amounts by the brain. The adrenal glands also produce progesterone, although adrenal progesterone is mainly used to make cortisol. Synthetic progestins like MPA (medroxyprogesterone acetate) do not fit into the same receptor "locks" as progesterone. MPA was developed specifically to prevent the buildup of the endometrial lining in women taking estrogens, and shares few other properties of progesterone. Only natural progesterone opens all the right hormone receptor locks.

Androgens and Androgen Precursors

Testosterone

In women, testosterone helps provide a sense of wellbeing, improves sex drive, and helps maintain vaginal mucosa and bone tissue. It is also involved in heart health, and maintenance of skin elasticity and muscle mass. Women have approximately 1/5 to 1/10 the amount of testosterone found in men, which explains why men have more muscle mass than women. Testosterone can be converted to estradiol via the enzyme aromatase. This conversion is particularly pronounced in women with a high percentage of body fat because aromatase is found in fat cells.

DHEA

Dehydroepiandrosterone (DHEA) is the most abundant steroid hormone in the body and is the principle androgen precursor. DHEA is produced by the adrenal glands and circulates in the blood primarily as the sulphate conjugate, DHEAS, which is a storage form of DHEA, just as estrone sulphate is for estrone. Figure 3 shows how DHEA can be used to make estradiol, estrone, estriol and testosterone.

Androstenedione

Androstenedione is made from DHEA in the adrenal glands. It is the building block for estrogens and testosterone and as such, is critical for the production of steroid hormones after menopause.

Glucocorticoids

Cortisol

Cortisol is released by the adrenal glands in response to physical and emotional stresses. Cortisol promotes the release of sugar into the blood, and plays an essential role in mobilizing the body's defenses against infection and inflammation. Cortisol levels are highest in the morning, to help the body combat the stress of overnight fasting and energize the body for the day's activities. Although not directly involved in the progression of menopause, cortisol is critically important in regulating the effects of other hormones.

HORMONE INTERACTIONS

The interactions between various hormone groups are as important as the actions of the hormones themselves. The interaction of cortisol with the various sex hormones shows how much of an impact stress can have on a woman's hormone balance. The following interactions involve cortisol:

Estrogens and Cortisol

Estrogens are derived from androstenedione and testosterone via the action of the enzyme aromatase. Cortisol stimulates aromatase activity, which in turn promotes estrogen formation. Cortisol also promotes deposition of fat around the waist, which is where the aromatase is! Simply put, excess cortisol translates into excess estrogens.

Progesterone and Cortisol

Progesterone interacts directly with cortisol at the receptor level. These two hormones can compete for the same receptor, like two people trying to fit through a doorway at once. If a woman is under considerable stress and producing a lot of cortisol, the cortisol may end up blocking the actions of progesterone. This is known as a functional deficiency. With a functional deficiency, progesterone levels may be normal, but the system *functions* as if there is too little, because high cortisol interferes with the actions of progesterone at the receptor site. Consequently, women under a lot of stress may need to supplement with progesterone.

DHEA and Cortisol

Cortisol and DHEA have opposite effects on immune function and regulation of blood sugar. For example, DHEA can improve sensitivity to insulin, which helps to lower blood glucose levels. Conversely, cortisol *increases* blood glucose levels. When cortisol levels are high, more DHEA must be released to balance the effects of the cortisol. Consequently, chronically elevated cortisol levels can result in a deficiency of DHEA. It is important when testing hormone levels to include both cortisol and DHEA (or its storage form, DHEA-sulphate) to get the full picture.

Androgens and Cortisol

The right *ratio* between cortisol and androgenic hormones is essential for maintaining muscle mass. Androgens help to build muscle, while cortisol breaks down muscle. As we age, we tend to have more cortisol relative to the androgens, resulting in a net loss of muscle mass and bone. The same imbalance can happen with chronic stress, and may contribute to premature aging. Cortisol and androgens can act on the same gene in opposite ways, so cortisol can directly oppose the message that the androgen is trying to deliver to cells. High cortisol levels can have the same effect on androgens as they have on progesterone. Specifically, having a high cortisol level can cause a functional androgen deficiency.

Thyroid and Cortisol

By now the picture should be clear: cortisol is a major player in the proper functioning of numerous hormones. This is especially true of thyroid hormone and cortisol. They have a mutually dependent relationship: a certain amount of thyroid is needed for cortisol to work properly, and a certain amount of cortisol is necessary for thyroid hormones to work properly. As a result, signs and symptoms of a deficiency in one hormone family can actually be due to a deficiency in the other family. Similarly, an excess of thyroid hormone can impair the activity of cortisol and vice versa.

There are many important interactions between hormones and maintaining the correct *balance* of the following hormones is essential to preventing or alleviating many common menopause symptoms:

Progesterone and Estrogens

It's no accident that estrogen and progesterone receptors are found in the same tissues. Progesterone and estrogens are like opposite ends of a seesaw. If they are in balance, the board is level. If a woman is too *heavy* in one hormone, the board slams into the ground on the heavy side. Women with an excess of estrogen over progesterone can experience a multitude of problems including weight gain at the hips, fluid retention, tender breasts, fibrocystic breasts, migraine headaches, and irritability to mention a few. Adding progesterone when there is an excess of estrogen normalizes ratio between estrogen and progesterone. Achieving the right balance of estrogen and progesterone can help prevent body fat build up, resolve fibrocystic breasts and breast tenderness, promote sleep, and exert a calming, mood-stabilizing effect. On the other hand, too much progesterone relative to estrogen can cause nausea, depression, drowsiness, foggy thinking and breast swelling, and can 'shut off' the effect of estrogens.

A complicating factor in maintaining the right balance between estrogens and progesterone is xenoestrogen pollution. Xenoestrogens are man-made chemicals (see inset page 21) that can fit into the estrogen receptor lock. Women with significant exposure to xenoestrogens may experience symptoms of estrogen excess even though their laboratory estrogen levels are normal.

Estrogens and Thyroid Hormones

There is close relationship between estrogens and thyroid hormone. Basically, excess estrogens suppress the action of thyroid hormone. Many women have normal thyroid tests but show signs and symptoms of low thyroid. This is called a functional deficiency. Progesterone can assist the action of thyroid hormones, and so excess estrogens, low progesterone and symptoms of low thyroid hormone often run together, while thyroid lab tests are usually normal.

XENOESTROGENS

Herbicides, pesticides and petroleum byproducts can act as xenoestrogens. They are very fat soluble, and consequently, accumulate readily in fatty tissues. Xenoestrogens also accumulate with each step up the food chain. Grains treated with herbicides are consumed by cattle and poultry, which in turn are consumed by humans. Dairy products are another common source of xenoestrogens. Petrochemical pollutants in the water contribute to xenoestrogen accumulation in fish. Storing and/or heating food in plastic containers is another potential source of xenoestrogens. Xenoestrogens have several possible effects on estrogen receptors:

- they may produce an estrogen effect
- they may cause more estrogen receptors to form
- they may inhibit the liver's ability to eliminate estrogens
- some can block the effect of estrogen at the receptor site

The net effect is increased estrogen exposure. There are some alarming health trends that may be due in part, to the prevalence of xenoestrogens:
- Hormone-dependent cancers have increased dramatically in the past several decades.
- Sperm counts have dropped by 50% since 1940
- Average onset of menstruation occurs a full two years earlier than it did just twenty years ago.

These are just a few signs that *something* is adversely affecting our hormonal health. The observed changes in hormone health follow closely on the heels of widespread use of herbicides, pesticides and petrochemicals. Perhaps it's just a coincidence, or perhaps not!

SUMMARY

The chemical messengers called hormones are an essential element of life; without hormones, the cells wouldn't know what to do, or when to do it! Non-human hormones don't have the same effects on all cells as naturally produced (bio-identical) hormones. Interactions between hormones are critical to all aspects of health, and imbalances can have serious health consequences.

Menopause symptoms are essentially a by-product of hormone imbalances brought about by a slowdown in ovarian function, compounded by other hormonal changes that accompany aging. In the next chapter we will take a closer look at the symptoms of menopause and to understand what these symptoms are trying to tell us about hormones and hormone balance.

CHAPTER THREE

What Is Menopause?

You know you're in menopause when the sound of sweat dripping on the floor keeps you awake at night! On the other hand, the *official* start of menopause is declared when a woman has gone twelve months without a menstrual period. On average this occurs around age fifty-one, but menopause can occur naturally anytime between ages forty and sixty. Premature menopause refers to menopause that occurs naturally before age forty. Menopause can also be artificially induced through radiation, surgical removal of both ovaries, or by chemical means.

Knowledge of hormone actions and interactions during menstruation is essential to understanding how hormone deficiencies and excesses can develop in menopause. Here's a brief discussion of the role of hormones in menstruation to help set the scene for discussion of the management of menopause symptoms.

THE MENSTRUAL CYCLE

No discussion of menopause would be complete without looking at the actions of hormones in the menstrual cycle. During menstruation, female sex hormones rise and fall with regularity, and there is a complex interaction between the hormone groups. The cessation of menses at the time of menopause fundamentally changes the rate and patterns of hormone release. There are a couple of ways of looking at the menstrual cycle. The first looks at the changes in hormone activity over an average 28-day cycle.

Follicular Phase

The follicular phase starts on day one, which is the first day of bleeding, and continues until just prior to ovulation, around day 13 or 14. During the follicular phase a number of follicles begin to *ripen* or mature. The ovaries contain as many as a million follicles at birth but only one follicle is selected each month to produce an ovum or egg. Rising levels of FSH (follicle stimulating hormone), secreted by the pituitary gland in the brain allow this one *dominant* follicle to develop. Levels of estradiol and estrone also start to rise. When the dominant follicle begins to develop around day 9, estradiol levels rise sharply and continue to rise until around day 13.

Ovulatory Phase

The estrogen peak near day 13 triggers the release of luteinizing hormone (LH), which stimulates the release of the egg from the dominant follicle. This is called ovulation. The purpose of ovulation is to release an egg for fertilization by sperm. The ovulatory phase lasts approximately 72 hours. Release of the egg from the dominant follicle signals the start of the luteal phase.

Luteal Phase

After the release of the egg, the dominant follicle is transformed into the corpus luteum. The corpus luteum is responsible for producing progesterone during the luteal phase. Progesterone levels rise sharply until about day 21. Estradiol and estrone levels also rise in the luteal phase, but to a lesser extent than earlier in the cycle. If fertilization doesn't occur, the levels of all three hormones start dropping around day 25 and menstruation is triggered to start on or about day 28. Figure 4 shows the levels of the various hormones as the menstrual cycle progresses.

Hormone Levels in the Menstrual Cycle

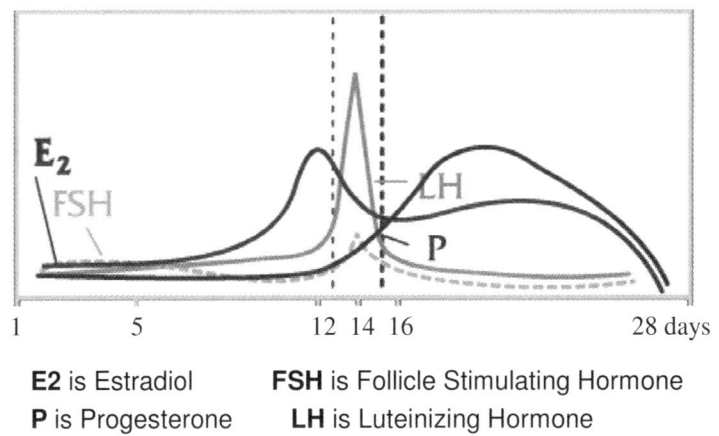

E2 is Estradiol		FSH is Follicle Stimulating Hormone	
P is Progesterone		LH is Luteinizing Hormone	

Figure 4

Proliferative and Secretory Phases

Another way of looking at the menstrual cycle is from the standpoint of the endometrium or lining of the uterus. In this view, a rough analogy to a house can be drawn. The

27

proliferative phase is the house *construction* phase in which the lining of the uterus, or endometrium is built up in preparation to receive a fertilized egg. After ovulation, the lining of the uterus changes under the influence of progesterone, in preparation to receive a fertilized egg. If fertilization doesn't occur, the lining of the uterus undergoes additional changes and is sloughed off or shed during menstruation. In other words, the house is *torn down* and the process starts over again.

PERI-MENOPAUSE

Peri-menopause literally means "around menopause" and refers to the years immediately preceding menopause. Changes in menstrual cycle regularity and/or the appearance of symptoms (see Table 1) generally signal the start of peri-menopause. The first signs that menopause is approaching often appear when a woman is in her forties. As women age, the number of viable ovarian follicles decreases. It becomes increasingly difficult to stimulate the remaining follicles to release an egg. Still, the body struggles to stimulate ovulation by increasing FSH and LH production. Occasionally, FSH and LH succeed in developing a follicle to maturity and ovulation occurs. However, as menopause nears, these attempts are increasingly ineffective and the ovaries begin to *sputter*. The second half of the cycle, the luteal phase, becomes shorter and menstrual periods become irregular as a result of repeated failures to ovulate. Missed ovulation leads to lower progesterone levels because no corpus luteum exists to produce progesterone.

Another feature of peri-menopause is that the body begins to produce more estradiol in the follicular phase (first half of the menstrual cycle). Failure to ovulate, a shortened luteal phase and higher estradiol levels in the follicular phase all add up to higher levels of estradiol relative to progesterone; a condition Dr. John Lee calls *estrogen dominance.*

As a result, symptoms of estrogen excess like headache, fluid retention and irritability frequently occur in peri-menopause. Declining estrogen and progesterone levels can change the frequency, length and intensity of menstrual periods. (Note: irregular periods and heavy bleeding can be signs of a more serious condition. Please contact your physician if you experience these symptoms.) The changes in hormone balance can result in a variety of symptoms. In the end, the few remaining follicles are too worn out to respond, and menstruation ceases entirely. The *change* has begun!

SYMPTOMS OF PERIMENOPAUSE

✦ Fatigue	✦ Irregular periods
✦ Less able to handle stress	✦ Fibrocystic breasts
✦ Weight gain	✦ Uterine fibroids
✦ Headaches	✦ Fluid retention
✦ Mood swings	✦ Depression
✦ Loss of sex drive	✦ Irritability

Table 1

AM I IN MENOPAUSE?

When women start to miss periods, they often wonder whether they're in menopause. In such cases, physicians sometimes check FSH and LH levels. Unfortunately these tests are notoriously unreliable. High levels of FSH and LH are signs the body is trying to stimulate ovulation, but these findings don't reveal whether or not the effort will be successful. If ovulation takes place, and progesterone is produced by the corpus luteum, then menstruation can occur. In other words, high levels of FSH and LH *may* be signs that a woman is close to menopause, but these levels may also be high in peri-menopausal women with irregular menstrual cycles. Many physicians mistakenly believe that FSH levels increase in response to low estrogen, and that a high FSH level indicates a need for estrogen supplementation. In fact, production of FSH is tied far more closely to a hormone called inhibin.

When ovulation stops altogether, estrogen and testosterone production drops and there is a general slow down of ovarian function. Since the corpus luteum is no longer formed, monthly production of progesterone ceases. The ovaries continue to produce small amounts of these hormones, but the adrenal glands become the principal source for post-menopausal hormones as outlined in the previous chapter. Many women do just fine with adrenally produced hormones, and do not experience debilitating symptoms of hormone deficiencies or imbalances. Others are not so fortunate.

HORMONE CHANGES IN MENOPAUSE
Estrogens

Despite the fact that estrogens are routinely prescribed for menopause, many women don't require them at all. In fact, some menopausal women are *estrogen dominant* and have too much estrogen relative to progesterone. Estrogen dominance can arise due to the drop in progesterone and accumulation of estrogen-like chemicals called xenoestrogens (see Chapter 2). In his book, *What Your Doctor May Not Tell You About Menopause*, Dr. John Lee lists a number of symptoms associated with estrogen dominance: loss of sex drive, depression, fatigue, fibrocystic breasts, foggy thinking, headaches, irritability, memory loss, and fluid retention. If any of these symptoms sound familiar, it could be because they're common symptoms of menopause. In other words, taking estrogen could make the symptoms of menopause worse for some women! The balancing effects of progesterone are key to resolving the issues of excess estrogen.

Conversely, there are symptoms that are clearly linked to a lack of estrogen. Vaginal dryness and incontinence are two common signs of estrogen deficiency. Brain fog and depression are also signs of a lack of estrogen, since the main estrogen, estradiol is needed to transport glucose into the brain. Without this fuel, the brain slows down. Sometimes adding a little progesterone can improve these symptoms, because progesterone makes the estrogen receptor more available to estrogen. Still, some women require small amounts of estrogen to relieve the symptoms associated with estrogen deficiency. This is more common in women who are slender, with a low percentage of body fat, since fat is the primary source of estrogens after menopause.

Progesterone

Production of progesterone drops dramatically at menopause. Other tissues still produce tiny amounts of progesterone but the major source, the ovarian corpus luteum, no longer exists. The abundance of xenoestrogens in our diets probably contributes to estrogen dominant/ progesterone deficient symptoms observed in menopause. Symptoms of progesterone deficiency parallel those of excess estrogen: loss of sex drive, depression, fatigue, fibrocystic breasts, foggy thinking, headaches, irritability, memory loss, and fluid retention. Normalizing the balance between progesterone and estrogens is essential to resolving these symptoms, and may even help prevent certain diseases from developing.

Androgens

Recall that testosterone is the principal androgen, and DHEA and androstenedione are androgen precursors. Androgen precursors are hormones on their way to becoming androgens (e.g. testosterone).

Testosterone

Testosterone levels can be significantly reduced in menopause if adrenal function is low. Low testosterone levels in women are associated with low sex drive, less physical pleasure from intercourse and a diminished sense of wellbeing. Restoring testosterone to normal levels often improves these symptoms. Normalizing testosterone levels may also prevent bone loss and increase bone density. The drop in testosterone at menopause can dramatically affect a woman's mood, sex drive and energy.

DHEA

Dehydroepiandrosterone (DHEA) deficiency is not associated with any accepted symptom pattern, but women with low baseline levels of DHEA sulphate reported an increased sense of wellbeing, decreased depression and anxiety, increased sex drive, and increased satisfaction with sex when given supplemental DHEA. Low levels of DHEA are also often associated with chronic health problems including chronic fatigue, hypertension and insulin resistance, as well as hypothyroidism. DHEA levels decline with age and for many women supplementation with DHEA restores energy, improves immune function and increases mental sharpness.

Androstenedione

Androstenedione deficiency results in lower levels of testosterone and estrogens since androstenedione is the primary source for postmenopausal production of these hormones. There are no recognized deficiency states associated specifically with androstenedione, but symptoms of estrogen and/or androgen deficiency are likely.

Cortisol

Cortisol production by the adrenal glands increases in response to stress. High cortisol levels are associated with numerous symptoms including weight gain, feeling 'tired but wired', memory problems, depression, and bone loss. This can lead to unstable blood glucose levels, fatigue, and increased susceptibility to infection. If the stress is severe enough, or lasts long enough, eventually the adrenal glands become depleted and fail to produce enough cortisol.

Depletion of the adrenal glands from chronic stress can result in inadequate production of cortisol, DHEA, and androstenedione. Low cortisol levels are associated with fatigue, low blood sugar, allergies, cold body temperature, aching muscles and poor exercise tolerance. Women who have had their ovaries removed are particularly at risk for repercussions from adrenal exhaustion as they are entirely dependent on the adrenals for hormone production.

Finding the Right Balance

Ovarian output of estradiol, progesterone and testosterone drops when a woman hits menopause and the adrenal glands become the primary source of these hormones. But, even women with significantly reduced levels of hormones, can glide through menopause without experiencing any unpleasant symptoms. What is it that separates the lucky from the unlucky? Clearly, the dwindling supply of hormones is only part of the story. As discussed in Chapter Two, maintaining a proper balance of hormones is also crucial. Too much of one hormone relative to another can lead to unpleasant symptoms. Knowing this, it should be common practice for the physician to investigate symptoms, look for imbalances and restore the balance. Clearly this hasn't been the experience of most women.

Lifestyle and dietary issues also contribute to menopause symptoms. Women with healthy adrenal glands, balanced hormones, a healthy diet, and an active lifestyle generally have the best experience of menopause. Having an accepting attitude about the aging process also helps to make menopause a positive experience. Christiane Northrup's book *The Wisdom of Menopause* is an excellent resource on the mental, emotional and spiritual aspects of menopause.

SUMMARY

Knowing that hormone excesses and deficiencies are common in menopause, it is likely that some women will need to rebalance their hormones with HRT. Studies like the WHIS have shown that not all HRT strategies are beneficial. The question is: where did hormone replacement go astray? One of the key issues is the type of hormones used. The next chapter looks at how the use of bio-identical hormones (identical to what the body produces naturally) differs from conventional HRT strategies. Chapter 4 also looks at when to use HRT, what mistakes were made in the past, and how we can learn from these mistakes and move forward.

CHAPTER FOUR

What Went Wrong With HRT?

For thousands of years physicians used treatments discovered by trial and error, and supported by anecdotes and general impressions. A given treatment continued in use because it stood the test of time, and was handed down from practitioner to trainee, generation after generation. In the past 10 to 15 years, there has been a steady push toward evidence-based medicine. In this model, everything the physician does, from diagnosis to treatment is supported by evidence, preferably in the form of large, randomized, placebo-controlled trials (RCTs). This is a laudable goal since it is estimated that only 20 to 30% of current medical practice is supported by evidence. There wasn't any evidence that oral horse estrogen was good for people when we started using it back in the 60's but we went ahead and used it anyway, and now there's a huge backlash against all hormone replacement therapies. Having said that, we must keep research and evidence-based medicine in perspective. Human beings are not one-size-fits-all creatures. Each woman is an individual, and hormone replacement therapies must reflect those individual variations. When evaluating hormone therapies, it is essential to consider the following:

The results of randomized trials may not be applicable to the general population

Trials have strict criteria for exclusion or participation; restrictions are placed on entry according to habits, medical history, medication use and other parameters. Patients however, don't fit neat patterns; they come in all shapes and sizes, with different histories. So no matter what the outcome of a controlled trial, practitioners still have to make judgment calls when they deal with patients one by one. Will the risks or benefits uncovered in a trial apply to *this* patient? Trials are supposed to reduce uncertainty, but for every question they answer, several new issues are raised. The notion that we can use clinical trials to achieve *perfect* medicine is naïve. In fact, RCTs are most helpful in determining the overall cost of a particular therapy to society. Unfortunately, this still leaves doubt as to whether any given individual will benefit.

Evidence should come from multiple sources

Evidence should be gathered from a variety of sources: large and small controlled human trials, uncontrolled human trials, anecdotal information, and studies on animals and cells. If the evidence consistently points to one conclusion, then there may be sufficient support for the therapy in question. Many different studies warned that the combination of MPA and conjugated estrogens increased the risks of heart disease and breast cancer. It wasn't necessary to wait ten years for the WHIS to *prove* it. Similarly, there is probably enough evidence to justify proceeding with other hormone replacement strategies. We aren't saying that the evidence is indisputable, but we are saying that there is enough for us to go on, if we proceed cautiously.

Conflicting results

"Recent study shows coffee is harmful/good for you"; "Vitamin C will save your life/increase your risk of cancer" and so on. The reality of research is that different studies of the same therapy can give opposite results unless all the critical factors have been isolated. Finding all the critical factors takes time, if it's even possible! Consequently, scientific findings often seem contradictory. Waiting for definitive answers on the *best* course of action for hormone replacement could take a very long time, or might never happen. Meanwhile, what should patients and their physicians do? Sometimes "nothing" and "wait and see" just aren't good enough.

Sources of funding for hormone research

Sadly, most physicians are unaware that there are more HRT options available than they learned about in medical school. The main reason for this knowledge gap is that bio-identical hormones are not easily patented. Pharmaceutical companies are interested in creating synthetic, patentable, look-alike hormones over which they have exclusive marketing rights. Critics of the WHIS questioned why natural progesterone was not included in the study, and the answer is simple: follow the money! Although the WHIS was conducted by the U.S. Government National Institute of Health, the medications were supplied by Wyeth-Ayerst, the pharmaceutical giant. It is highly unlikely that an unbiased, large scale trial of bio-identical hormone replacement options will ever be undertaken, due to pharmaceutical industry influence and funding issues.

The goal of hormone replacement was to help women live longer and healthier, but the main conclusion of the WHIS was that the combination of oral conjugated equine estrogen and MPA won't help women achieve either of those goals. So after 40 years of large-scale hormone tinkering, it's back to square one. Or is it? Bio-identical hormone replacement therapy (BHRT) has been criticized for its lack of long-term studies, but there are many good sized (up to several hundred women), well-conducted studies of one to two-year's duration looking at the effects of oral estriol, and oral micronized progesterone. Bear in mind that there are *no* long-term studies showing that *any* other hormone replacement strategies are completely safe. The evidence for BHRT is by no means irrefutable, but it seems to be pointing in a positive direction. To understand why BHRT might be a better option, it's important to understand how bio-identical hormones differ from hormones used in conventional hormone replacement

BIO-IDENTICAL HORMONES

Hormones are powerful and affect every tissue in our bodies, directly or indirectly. Since there isn't a complete blueprint available for the body, we don't know exactly which doors (hormone receptors) need to stay closed and which doors need to be open. Some doors open and close as the occupants come and go. When it comes to hormones, it isn't smart to padlock some doors and wedge others wide open by forcing non-human hormones on the system. It makes for an unhappy household. Opening the bathroom door when someone is inside is liable to cause some screeching! In a similar fashion, the high incidence of side effects with combined Premarin®/Provera® is the body's way of signaling its distress. Unfortunately, these cries of distress appear to have been drowned out by the need to sell more pharmaceuticals.

Estrogens

Conventional hormone replacement commonly uses estrogens extracted from pregnant mare's urine (conjugated equine estrogens or Premarin®). Although approximately half of the estrogen extracted from the urine of pregnant mares is identical to human estrogens, there are dozens, if not hundreds of non-human hormones and hormone by-products present. Many of these compounds persist in the body for weeks or months, because human beings aren't equipped to break down horse hormones. This may cause harm over the long term. We don't feed cat food to fish, and we don't give birdseed to dogs, so why would we give horse hormones to people?

Since the first edition of this book was published, the results of the Premarin® only arm of the WHIS have been released. It is worth discussing these findings in more detail, as they add to our knowledge of HRT. In a nutshell, the WHIS showed that the combination of Premarin® and

THE WOMEN'S HEALTH INITIATIVE STUDY (WHIS) Key Points
Premarin® only arm

THE STUDY
- ≈ 11,000 hysterectomized women
- Age range: 50-79 years
- 0.625 mg Premarin vs placebo
- 6.8 years of follow-up
- Terminated 1 year early
- 3 to 4% dropout rate for both active and placebo

RESULTS
- The study was stopped early because it was determined that no new information on HRT and disease prevention would be forthcoming if the trial were allowed to go to completion
- Compared to placebo, Premarin® caused:
  - 40% more strokes
  - No change in heart disease risk
  - No change or possible decrease in breast cancer risk
  - Possible increase in blood clots
  - Possible increase in risk of Alzheimer's Dementia
  - 40% *fewer* hip fractures

Overall, this arm of the WHIS proved that oral dosing with Premarin® alone was less harmful to women than Premarin® plus Provera®, but more harmful than placebo.

Provera® clearly increased the risks of heart disease, breast cancer, stroke, blood clots and dementia. In contrast, with Premarin® alone, only the risk of stroke increased significantly, while the risk of blood clots and dementia increased slightly. In the final analysis, it seems that much (but not all) of the 'bad rap' attributed to HRT was due to Provera®.

This latest information from the WHIS is consistent with our view of receptor-hormone interactions. Synthetic hormones like Provera® appear to be the real 'bad actors' in HRT, because they don't fit the receptor *lock* in the same way as natural hormones. Human hormones are the right *key* for the receptor *lock*, and therefore open the right *doors*. Because conjugated equine estrogens contain some human estrogens along with non-human horse estrogens, at least some of the right *doors* will get opened. So, it is not surprising that the Premarin® only arm was less harmful than Premarin® plus Provera®.

Nevertheless, there is still a substantial risk of stroke associated with oral Premarin®, and it is important not to lose sight of that fact. There are several reasons why oral Premarin® alone might significantly increase risk of strokes:

➤ Firstly, Premarin® contains estrogens from another species, and non-human hormones do not have the same effect on receptors as bio-identical human hormones.

➤ Secondly, women are probably taking much higher doses of estrogen than necessary, due to the inefficiency of oral delivery.

➤ And finally, taking Premarin® orally disturbs the natural pattern of proteins, such as clotting factors, which are made by the liver. Enhanced clotting directly increases stroke risk.

An in-depth discussion of the disadvantages of taking estrogens orally occurs later in this chapter.

From the WHIS we also know that giving oral conjugated equine estrogens alone does not increase breast cancer risk. In fact, the Premarin®only arm of the study showed a slight *decrease* in the risk of breast cancer over the seven-year study. On the surface, this might seem surprising since we have been conditioned to believe that estrogens cause breast cancer. The fact is that the right amount of estrogen is probably good for the breasts, just as the right amount of estrogen is good for tissues of the vagina and bladder. Breast cancer risk increases when too much estrogen is given and when estrogen is given in combination with synthetic progestins like Provera.®

At the end of the day, the WHIS tells us that hormone replacement therapy is not all bad; it simply heightens our awareness of the importance of using the right hormones in the right dose, and delivering them in the right way. Giving bio-identical hormones in the minimum dose required to prevent symptoms, and delivering them through the skin upholds the lessons learned from the WHIS.

There are numerous human hormone products available commercially, some of which are ideally suited for the purposes of bio-identical hormone replacement therapy. Chapter 7 and Appendix A go into more detail on available bio-identical hormone products. Estradiol, estrone and estriol are naturally produced estrogens that are commonly used in BHRT. Human bio-identical hormones are not the enemy of human tissue if they are used in appropriate amounts and delivered in a natural fashion.

Estradiol

Since estradiol is the principle hormone produced by the ovaries prior to menopause, it is an excellent choice for BHRT. The body is used to taking estradiol and transforming it into other hormones as needed. Research on estradiol clearly shows it has positive effects on bone, blood vessels, cells lining the vaginal wall, skin and bladder. As far as the effects of estrogen on the brain go, there was a slight (though not statistically significant) increase in Alzheimer's dementia in the Premarin® only arm of the WHIS. However, previous research suggested estradiol was protective to the brain. The fact that Premarin® contains non-human estrogens along with estradiol, may explain why the WHIS showed no benefit to the brain from Premarin® use.

Estrone

Much of the estradiol produced naturally in the body is converted to estrone. Estrone in turn can be made into a storage form called estrone sulphate. One feature of breast cancer cells is that they tend to accumulate large amounts of estrone sulphate, which can be converted back to estrone and then on to estradiol as needed. In other words, estrone sulphate acts like slow-release fertilizer for estrogen-sensitive breast cancer cells. In fact, sulphatase inhibitors, drugs that block the conversion of estrone sulphate to estrone, are being studied as treatments for breast cancer.

Furthermore, there is mounting evidence that a metabolite (breakdown product) of estrone called 4-hydroxyestrone plays a role in the initiation of breast cancer. Overdosing women with estrone might lead to an accumulation of higher than normal levels of potential cancer promoting estrone by-products like estrone sulphate and 4-hydoxyestrone, which can be carcinogenic under the wrong circumstances (e.g. in combination with synthetic progestins like Provera®). Clearly, it is sensible to avoid giving excess estrone. Some women, in particular those with little body fat, may need to supplement with small amounts of estrone, if their measured levels are low. In most women however, there is probably no role for estrone supplementation because of concerns about accumulation of estrone sulphate, 4-hydroxyestrone and their potential impact on breast cancer cell growth.

Because estrone sulphate is the most abundant estrogen and the major storage form of estrogen in the body, measurement of this hormone in saliva or blood will likely be useful in determining a woman's overall estrogen status. In other words, this measurement could be used to determine whether a woman is taking too much estrogen, or to decide whether *any* estrogen should be prescribed. Estrone sulphate may also be a useful marker for breast cancer risk. In theory, women with larger stores of estrogen could have a greater risk of developing breast cancer.

Estriol

The use of estriol is controversial for many physicians, in part because estriol isn't manufactured by pharmaceutical companies and also because it isn't discussed in medical schools, except in the context of its role in pregnancy. Consequently, it's important to examine the evidence for estriol in more detail.

Estriol has been widely used in North America for the past 15 to 20 years and in Europe for even longer. It has been widely researched in Europe, Japan and to a lesser extent, North America. It is clear from this research that estriol has estrogenic effects. Estriol relieves hot flashes, lowers cholesterol, relieves vaginal dryness, restores normal vaginal bacterial counts, and may offer relief from recurrent urinary tract infections. There is also evidence that estriol helps dilate blood vessels as estradiol does. There is no firm evidence that estriol alone builds bone.

Many researchers are interested in estriol because it doesn't stimulate thickening of the endometrium to the same extent as estradiol and estrone. A one-year study of estriol alone, showed no significant difference in the thickness of the endometrium between estriol and placebo users. However, the estriol group had a tendency toward more non-cancerous growths (polyps) than the placebo group. Increased mammographic breast density is considered to be a risk factor for breast cancer. A study comparing estriol to other estrogens showed that estriol caused the least increase in breast density, although it still caused a slight increase in breast density. These findings reinforce the fact that *no estrogen* should be administered without progesterone to oppose it, and careful attention should be paid to the dose used.

Recall from Figures 2 and 3 that estriol is at the end of the estrogen pathway: estradiol is converted to estrone and estrone can then convert into estriol. For the most part, estriol stays as estriol, although some tissues (the uterus in particular) can convert estriol back to other estrogens. Since it generally doesn't convert to anything else when it is swallowed, estriol can be given orally with confidence.

If we're trying to stay as close to natural hormone levels as possible, does the use of estriol even fit into bio-identical hormone replacement? After all, estriol levels are only high when a woman is pregnant, so why would we give estriol to women in menopause? Some researchers have suggested that high estriol levels are nature's way of protecting the fetus from the mother's estradiol. High levels of estriol relative to estradiol block the access of estradiol to its receptors. Pregnancy is protective against breast cancer, and estriol may play an important role in this protective effect. In rats, giving estriol along with a known breast carcinogen decreased the risk of breast cancer. So, there are a number of indicators that estriol is probably a safe choice for bio-identical hormone replacement.

In North America, estriol is usually combined with estradiol and sometimes with estrone. The estradiol/estriol combination is called BiEst and the combination of estradiol/estriol/estrone is known as TriEst (see Appendix A). Given the possible association between estrone sulphate, 4-hydroxyestrone and breast cancer, it makes more sense to use BiEst, and avoid estrone accumulation. To date though, there have been no human trials of TriEst or BiEst. The lack of research specifically on BiEst and TriEst products has made many practitioners wary of these combinations. They say they are unproven. In fact, as previously detailed there are many small, one and two year trials of estriol alone. Adding a small amount of estradiol offers the benefits of estrogens, while maintaining the potential protective effects of estriol.

Progesterone

Somewhere between studying undergraduate biochemistry and completing their medical training, some doctors develop a kind of amnesia regarding progesterone. Physicians learn about its role in the menstrual cycle and that progesterone is essential for pregnancy, but somehow the critical *differences* between progesterone and synthetic progestins are forgotten. Examples of progestins include MPA (medroxyprogesterone acetate), norethindrone acetate, and levonorgestrel. Progestin is actually a made-up word that refers to a class of drugs that has the same effect on the endometrium as progesterone. Progestins do not have the same effects as progesterone on all tissues. For example, progesterone is vital to pregnancy, but the progestins are considered harmful in pregnancy. Even to a layperson, this should suggest that progestins are not the same as progesterone! Unfortunately, many health professionals and researchers still use the terms progesterone and progestin interchangeably.

The careless, or not-so-careless interchange of these terms lulled the medical community into thinking that the synthetic progestin MPA was as good as bio-identical progesterone for many years. This probably did more harm to the cause of hormone replacement than any other factor. There are various large HRT studies that have used the synthetic progestin MPA and demonstrated that the risks significantly outweighed the benefits! The combination of MPA and oral estrogen increases the risk of breast cancer over and above the risk of oral estrogen alone. The WHIS and other studies before it showed that the combination of oral estrogens and MPA also increases the risk of heart disease. This is not new information. MPA counteracts the beneficial blood vessel dilating effects of estradiol, in both animals and humans. Progesterone does *not* interfere with the vasodilating effects of estradiol. MPA given alone also increases the risk of blood clots. Progesterone has little effect on C-reactive protein, a marker of inflammation linked to heart disease, while MPA *elevates* C-reactive protein. Progesterone slows the overgrowth of arterial smooth muscle cells, a step in the development of heart disease, while MPA promotes this overgrowth of cells.

In retrospect, MPA was probably the worst possible partner for estrogen. Of course pharmaceutical companies have developed other progestins, and more are on the way. To be fair, some of the newer progestins (e.g. norethindrone acetate) don't seem to have the same negative effects on the heart and blood vessels as MPA. Nevertheless, the dramatic differences between MPA and progesterone show it is much more sensible to stick to the original blueprint and use only bio-identical hormones for hormone replacement therapy.

So why hasn't natural progesterone received more attention? For many years, the consensus was that progesterone couldn't be absorbed orally. This issue was solved by micronizing, or grinding the progesterone very finely, to increase the area available for absorption. Various studies have shown that oral micronized progesterone *does* stabilize and protect the uterine endometrium from estrogen. The most recent study of this kind was the PEPI trial, in which oral micronized progesterone was compared head to head with MPA, along with oral estrogen. Women who received progesterone had less breakthrough bleeding than those who received MPA, and there was no difference in the rates of uterine cancer between the two groups.

In 2003, a three-month study of oral micronized progesterone (Prometrium®) in postmenopausal women concluded that this form of progesterone has no negative impact on important indicators of heart disease like blood pressure, cholesterol, or the ability of the arteries to dilate.

There are numerous commercially available human hormone products, some of which are ideally suited for the purposes of BHRT. We'll go through these products in more detail in Chapter 7 on restoring the balance of hormones. The key point to remember is that human bio-identical hormones are not the enemy of human tissue. It's all a question of keeping them in balance, giving the right amounts and *delivering* them in the right way.

HORMONE DELIVERY SYSTEMS

Any therapy aimed at replacing hormones should try to approximate the natural daily ebb and flow of the hormone in question. The ovaries don't make a full pot of estradiol every morning; they produce a fairly steady drip through the day. Estradiol replacement therapy should therefore probably be given in the same way: slow release into the system. The level of testosterone is typically higher in the morning and declines through the day, and replacement therapy should also attempt to achieve a higher level first thing in the morning. It's also important to remember that hormone levels change *throughout* the menstrual cycle. Progesterone, for example, is highest in the luteal phase (second half) of the menstrual cycle, so use of progesterone prior to menopause should reflect this trend. The body has a natural break from significant hormone exposure during menstruation, and this break is worth replicating when giving hormone replacement therapy. Not all women need the break, but for some it makes a big difference. Exposure to the same dose of hormone every day may cause receptors to stop listening to messages being delivered by the hormones. This is called receptor down-regulation and can reduce the effectiveness of hormone therapy.

What's the best way to mimic natural hormone release and distribution? Are hormones best taken orally, or is there another way that's closer to natural delivery? The most commonly used hormone delivery systems are oral and transdermal (through the skin). A discussion of the properties of each follows. Appendix A goes into more detail on the specifics of bio-identical hormones and all the hormone delivery options available to women.

Oral Delivery

Any hormone or drug we *swallow* is modified by the gut and delivered to the liver *before* going to the heart and tissues. The gut and liver change most of the hormone they receive into more water-soluble conjugate forms for easier elimination from the body. Therefore, if the aim is to deliver hormones to the body as naturally as possible, delivery through the skin is best. Skin delivery and ovarian delivery of hormones are not exactly the same, but their differences are small compared to the differences between oral and ovarian delivery. A discussion of oral administration of hormones is necessary to be able to understand the advantages of delivery through skin.

Estrogens

It is easy to be fooled when giving estrogens orally. Many doctors and pharmacists mistakenly believe only 10% of an oral dose of estrogen is absorbed; they think the other 90% goes immediately into the toilet. In fact, almost all of an oral dose of estrogen is used by the body. Consider this: a doctor learns in medical school that only 10% of an estradiol pill is available to tissue. So she thinks that if she gives someone a 2 mg estradiol pill, she is really only giving that person 10% of the labeled dose, or 0.2 mg of estradiol. Wrong! She is giving that person 2 mg of estrogen, but only 10% stays as estradiol. The extra 1.8 mg is still present, but it is in the form of estrogen byproducts or metabolites. Research in the 1980's showed that more than half of estradiol or estrone swallowed is changed to estrone sulphate. Estrone sulphate is a *storage* form of estrogen, and as such can be used to feed estrogen dependent breast cancer cells. Therefore, women must only be given enough estrogen to meet their immediate needs. Hormone replacement should not increase the level of stored estrogen beyond what is normally present before menopause. As mentioned previously, a good way to gauge whether a woman is overdosed on estrogen might be to measure estrone sulphate levels.

Many studies have shown that oral estrogen, at least in the doses used in the past, affects the natural patterns of liver protein production. These proteins are involved in blood clotting, regulation of insulin, and delivery of thyroid hormone and cortisol to tissue. Therefore, giving estrogens orally could theoretically result in an increased tendency to clotting, poor insulin regulation and decreased thyroid function. The WHIS confirmed this, as Premarin® given orally alone was shown to increase the risk of stroke and blood clots.

We mentioned that only 10% of an oral dose of estradiol stays as estradiol, and that over half the dose winds up as estrone sulphate. A substantial amount of the remaining *unaccounted for* oral estradiol dose turns into estrone. Whenever we supplement with oral estradiol or estrone, an excess of estrone relative to estradiol occurs. This disturbs the normal balance between these two hormones. For example, before menopause, a woman has one to two times as much estradiol as estrone in her blood (estradiol: estrone ratio >1). After menopause a woman has *less* estradiol than estrone (estradiol to estrone ratio between 0.3 and 0.5). When a postmenopausal woman is given oral estradiol or estrone, this ratio goes even lower. If hormone replacement is supposed to make women feel younger, why move *away* from the balance of hormones found prior to menopause? Giving estradiol or estrone orally upsets the balance between these two hormones and results in a blood hormone profile more like that of an older woman.

It would seem then that many of the estrogen replacement problems in the past stem from oral estrogen supplementation. When we swallow estrogens, we don't get the natural pattern of estrogen breakdown products we want, we give 10 times more estrogen than is necessary and we disturb the liver. (The exception is estriol, which cannot be readily broken down into any other estrogens.)

Progesterone

The situation regarding oral progesterone is similar to that of oral estrogens: about 90% of the progesterone we swallow is converted into progesterone by-products or metabolites. The body makes around 20 to 25 mg of progesterone/day during the two weeks before menstruation. The usual dose of oral micronized progesterone averages around 200 mg per day, which delivers about 20 mg of unchanged progesterone into the bloodstream. Unlike oral estrogens however, the metabolites of oral progesterone don't appear to be harmful. Many of them have sedative properties, and this can be used to advantage. For example, women experiencing problems with anxiety and insomnia often experience relief after taking progesterone orally. Some of these same metabolites are also produced naturally during pregnancy when the progesterone level is high, and this leads to the well-known third trimester mellowing of mood.

Delivery Through the Skin

Humans have known for thousands of years that the skin is very effective for delivering medicines. In fact, you could say that poultices were the original skin *patches*. Delivery through skin allows any hormone or drug absorbed into skin blood vessels to go directly to the heart for distribution to all tissues, with the exception of skin on the abdomen. (Hormones applied there go straight to the liver). Hormones made in the ovaries and adrenal glands also pass directly into the blood, travel to the heart and back out to all the other tissues of the body, bypassing the liver for the most part. Therefore, if the aim is to deliver hormones to the body in as natural a fashion as possible, delivery through skin appears to be the best option. In fact, the evidence in favour of transdermal delivery of hormones is steadily accumulating

Dosing with estradiol patches ranges from 25 micrograms (0.025 mg) to 100 micrograms per day. For compounded creams, the average estradiol dose is around 100 to 200 micrograms (0.1 to 0.2 mg) per day. Just 50 micrograms estradiol daily delivered via patch has been shown to build bone and relieve hot flashes whereas it takes at least 500 micrograms (0.5 mg) of oral estradiol to do the same. Also, transdermal delivery of estrogens doesn't appear to have the negative effects on liver proteins that oral estrogens do. Oral estrogens increase the tendency to form blood clots, while transdermal estradiol has no effect on clotting.

Estradiol is very efficiently delivered through the skin, and this is also true for progesterone, despite what is commonly believed. Of all the steroid hormones, progesterone is the most fat soluble, and consequently is the *most* likely steroid hormone to be absorbed through the skin. In fact, a paper presented at the 2004 annual meeting of the American Society for Clinical Pharmacology and Therapeutics showed conclusively that the same amount of progesterone was delivered to the blood over 24 hours whether the progesterone was swallowed (200 mg per day) or rubbed on the skin (40 mg twice daily).

Another study showed that application of progesterone to the skin of rats resulted in the accumulation of progesterone in lung, salivary gland, brain and uterine tissue. In particular, the level in the uterus was *eight times* that measured in the blood. And, a one-year study of progesterone cream in 43 women showed that it is more effective than placebo for the relief of hot flashes. Clearly, progesterone cream has demonstrable benefits for women.

Nevertheless, concern is often expressed that progesterone may not protect against endometrium build-up, and therefore women may be at greater risk of endometrial cancer. A twenty-woman study looking at this issue was published in 2003. It examined the effects of progesterone cream or MPA (Provera®) on the endometrium of women taking Premarin®. The study concluded that after six months of cither therapy, there was no difference in the endometrial biopsies obtained. In other words, progesterone was just as effective as MPA (Provera®) at protecting the endometrium. Dr. Helene Leonetti, one of the authors of that study, is an obstetrician-gynecologist who has used progesterone cream in over 3000 patients and reports that it is safe, well-tolerated and effective in the prevention of uterine cancer and overgrowth of the uterine endometrium. A study published in 1995 found that progesterone cream applied to the breasts along with estradiol effectively suppressed the stimulation of breast cells seen with estradiol alone. These studies, and numerous others, confirm the fact that progesterone cream is well absorbed through the skin and has meaningful effects on tissue.

Other means of delivering progesterone to the body include vaginal suppositories and vaginal gels. Vaginal gel delivery results in sustained high blood levels of progesterone, without the conversion to progesterone metabolites seen with oral progesterone. Progesterone has also been delivered as a nasal spray, where just 30 mg/day had the same effect as 200 mg of oral progesterone. Studies consistently demonstrate that progesterone is readily absorbed through various sites including the skin, the vagina and even the mucous membranes in the nose.

Even though there hasn't been a ten-year, 16,000 person study of progesterone cream, there are multiple lines of evidence indicating that progesterone cream is well absorbed and is successfully delivered to tissue. The main concern with progesterone cream is whether or not it is able to prevent overgrowth of endometrial tissue when given in combination with estrogen. There is no clear-cut evidence yet, but as mentioned previously, rat studies show that progesterone levels in the uterus do rise significantly with application of progesterone cream.

Many women use wild yam cream believing that it offers the same benefits as progesterone cream. In fact, the components of wild yam do *not* convert to progesterone in the body. Confusion probably stems from the fact that some progesterone cream manufacturers use wild yams as a starting point to chemically manufacture progesterone, and some wild yam creams have had progesterone added to them in manufacturing. In the final analysis, wild yam cream does not work the same as progesterone cream, and only creams with progesterone in them have all the benefits of progesterone.

Many practitioners are concerned about the variable quality of progesterone formulations. Progesterone cream is available without a prescription in the United States and some of these *over-the-counter* (OTC) creams find their way into Canada. Analysis has shown that some have *no* progesterone in them, but others are of very high quality and have been used successfully by thousands of women. The quality of prescription hormone creams can vary as well, depending on the knowledge and skill of the pharmacist (Appendix A - BHRT Products). It is best to deal with a pharmacist that specializes in prescription compounding (see Resources).

HORMONE DOSES

Recall that oral estrogens are well absorbed, but that only 10% of what you swallow stays in its original form. The rest is changed to other estrogens like estrone sulphate. Unfortunately, breast cancer cells accumulate estrone sulphate, and use it to feed breast tumors. It therefore follows that the *minimum* dose of estradiol or estrone should be used to relieve symptoms and restore hormone balance, in order to minimize formation of excess estrone and estrone sulphate. Delivering estradiol through skin, and giving the lowest effective dose helps to reduce the risks associated with estrogen replacement.

Flexibility of hormone dosing options is also important. Research indicates that compliance with HRT increases when women have the option of choosing from a range of delivery systems and doses. Custom bio-identical hormone formulations provided by compounding pharmacists offer this flexibility, as doses can usually easily be changed by fractions of a milligram.

WHY SUPPLEMENT HORMONES?

Isn't hormone replacement a contradiction? After all it *is* natural for hormone levels to drop after menopause. Our great-grandparents never used hormone replacement, and they managed. Why should we interfere? Why not let nature take its course? Well, women *should* do everything possible to maintain hormone balance naturally by eating healthfully, exercising, avoiding toxins and taking appropriate herbs and supplements. But even women who do all the right things can end up needing hormone replacement. Our environment and food supplies are very different from what they were centuries ago. In general, women now consume fewer plant foods (and therefore fewer plant hormones) and more man-made chemicals than previous generations. Women today also experience different stresses and have a more hectic lifestyle with less sleep, nutritionally depleted foods, too much caffeine, and not enough relaxation. This can contribute to adrenal exhaustion. Some women have had hysterectomies or other hormone-altering surgeries and no longer make enough sex hormones. If hormone supplementation can help restore the balance, then why should women suffer unnecessarily?

Unfortunately, only an enlightened minority pays attention to the *balance* of hormones. Few doctors monitor hormone levels and, even if they do, most only measure serum estradiol or progesterone levels. Estradiol is only one piece of the estrogen puzzle, and estradiol levels don't reflect the accumulation of estrone sulphate. Serum progesterone doesn't measure just progesterone, it also captures the progesterone metabolites. As a result, serum progesterone levels may not reflect the *actual* balance between estrogens and progesterone. Chapter 6 has a thorough discussion of the importance of hormone testing in monitoring and restoring hormone balance.

Many researchers and physicians believe the best hormone replacement strategy is to give hormones in a natural, commonsense way that is in tune with body processes and rhythms. Jonathan Wright, a respected natural medicine pioneer, once commented that visitors from another planet would probably express astonishment at the notion that we would give ourselves estrogens from another species. Dr. Wright also dared to suggest that we follow the natural template that has been in place for as many years as human beings have walked the earth. In other words, give human hormones to humans; deliver them so they are metabolized in the same way as if they were homegrown; keep the right balance of hormones, and above all, don't give hormone doses in excess of what the body requires!

Early in 2004, Suzanne Somers' book *The Sexy Years* was published. Ms. Somers has done women a great service by raising the general level of awareness about BHRT. The attention her book received has empowered many women to seek help for their hormone issues. However, one issue arising from Ms. Somers' interview with Dr. Schwarzbein (Chapter Five of *The Sexy Years*) is her claim that women need to have periods while they are on hormones.

Dr. Schwarzbein makes the argument that women should continue to have periods in menopause, because not having periods mimics pregnancy, and pregnancy is associated with health risks. Our position is that there is a sound biological reason why women in menopause do not have periods. Menopause is the time of life when the body gets a rest from long-term exposure to estrogens. It is understood that women who have never given birth, or who have their first child late in life, have a greater risk of breast cancer because of their prolonged exposure to estrogens from continual periods. Although Dr. Schwarzbein suggests that pregnant women have a higher risk of breast cancer, there is clear evidence to the contrary. A 2004 paper titled *Breast cancer: the protective effect of pregnancy* states: "It has been firmly established in epidemiological studies that early full-term pregnancy affords lifetime protection against the development of breast cancer." The protection against breast cancer offered by pregnancy may be reduced if the woman is insulin resistant (see inset), but pregnancy does not cause insulin resistance, high refined carbohydrate diets are the likely main culprit.

INSULIN RESISTANCE

Insulin is a hormone secreted in response to a glucose rise in the bloodstream. Glucose is produced by the breakdown of food, and large amounts of refined carbohydrates quickly result in high glucose levels. With insulin resistance, the levels of insulin remain high because the tissues are not responding to the message insulin is trying to deliver. Prolonged high levels of insulin can result in increased fat storage, and may increase risk of diabetes and cancer in women.

High levels of DHEAS and testosterone are often found in women who are insulin resistant.

In the final analysis, it is *not normal* for women in their fifties to be bleeding regularly. Making women have periods into their fifties and sixties means giving them enough estrogen to thicken the lining of the uterus to stimulate bleeding (shedding of the endometrium). Why give more estrogen and potentially increase breast cancer risk at a time of life when the risk is already high? The rational approach is to give the smallest dose of estrogens needed to relieve symptoms. We should not be aiming to turn sixty year olds into twenty year olds. Women's bodies were not designed to have periods beyond age fifty, and we need to respect that and not try to duplicate hormone conditions of the reproductive years.

Dr Schwarzbein also claims that a break in therapy is needed each month, as continuous (no break) Premarin® plus Provera® stresses the adrenal glands. In fact, standard BHRT practice is consistent with Dr. Schwarzbein's recommendations, because a five to seven day 'holiday' from progesterone and estrogens each month is recommended to maintain tissue sensitivity to these hormones. The real difference in our philosophies is the amount of hormone given. Dr. Schwarzbein prescribes larger hormone doses to produce a withdrawal bleed (a period), while we advocate the smallest possible dose to resolve symptoms. In particular, the high doses of estrogens required to cause a withdrawal bleed are likely to increase stores of estrone sulphate. As previously discussed, estrone sulphate may act as a kind of 'fertilizer' for breast cancer cells. We believe there is ample evidence that giving higher than necessary doses of estrogens may be harmful.

Ultimately though, the point of BHRT is to help women to feel better, and do it safely and effectively. The following are common rationales for bio-identical hormone replacement therapy:

(1) **Short term BHRT (less than 5 years) to ease the passage through early menopause.** Short-term BHRT appears to be well tolerated, and provides relief for menopausal symptoms. However, if the length of therapy is restricted to just 2 or 3 years, then conventional HRT, with its reasonably well defined risks and benefits, may also be an acceptable option for some women and their physicians.

(2) **Long term BHRT (more than 10 years) to make up for potential hormone deficiencies introduced by gynecologic surgery (i.e hysterectomy and/or oophorectomy).** Note that even if the ovaries remain, they often fail within a few months or years of removal of the uterus. Women who have their ovaries removed before menopause age faster, and are at increased risk of heart disease and bone loss if hormones are not replaced.

(3) **Long term (more than 10 years), post-menopausal BHRT aimed at improving health, and reducing the burden of chronic illnesses such as heart disease, osteoporosis and dementia.** Although the evidence for long term BHRT is far from clear-cut, there are tantalizing clues that bio-identical hormones *should* help prevent heart disease, bone loss and dementia after menopause. If something is safe for the long term, it will also be safe in the short term. Unfortunately there

are currently no studies supporting the long-term safety of *any* hormone replacement strategy.

SUMMARY

Many scientists and physicians today feel that science is all-knowing, can improve on nature, and that we can play around at will with hormone systems that are almost unimaginably complex and interwoven. What about the *common-sense* bio-identical hormone replacement approach that is *not* taught to medical students? This approach is rejected as being unscientific, but actually is much more logical than trying to forcefully insert synthetic and non-human hormones into a complex, delicate web. The WHIS was supposed to show women how to live longer and healthier with HRT, but instead showed that combined conjugated equine estrogen and MPA clearly contradict that goal. Unfortunately this has made many women and their physicians suspicious of any type of hormone replacement.

We are at an impasse with hormone replacement. Most health professionals feel that the only way around this impasse is to either walk away from the whole concept for now and wait (potentially in vain) for more evidence, or accept the post-WHIS spin-doctoring and continue giving the same drugs but with more restrictions. There is another option though: to look at the whole picture from a fresh angle, reasoning from first principles. This is the reasoning behind bio-identical hormone replacement therapy. The evidence for BHRT is not bullet-proof. We don't know that BHRT will be 100% safe for every woman, over her entire postmenopausal lifespan. However, common sense coupled with the evidence accumulated so far, suggests that bio-identical hormones delivered in ways that closely mimic natural patterns and rhythms will, in the long run, prove to be safer and more effective than anything we discover by tinkering in the lab.

PART TWO

3 Simple Steps

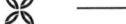

1) **Symptom Assessment**

2) **Uncovering Imbalances with Hormone Testing**

3) **Restoring Hormone Balance**

CHAPTER FIVE

STEP 1
Symptom Assessment

In the last chapter, we discussed reasons for considering bio-identical hormone replacement, for both short-term and long-term use. Many women wonder whether it's really necessary to take anything for menopause if annoying symptoms are their only complaint. The answer is another question; "How annoying are the symptoms?" For many women, the symptoms associated with hormone decline in menopause are life altering, making it difficult to manage their days and their lives. In such cases, some form of hormone intervention is a necessity. Women don't need to suffer in silence. Hormone imbalances may also contribute to chronic illness, so it's better to look at the symptoms and try to nip hormone problems in the bud *before* a chronic illness develops.

Symptoms can be associated with deficiencies or excesses of each of the four main categories of steroid hormones: estrogens, progesterone, androgen and androgen precursors, and glucocorticoids (specifically: cortisol). Assessment of these symptoms, along with hormone testing, is an excellent way to determine hormone issues. The cancellation of the combined Premarin®/Provera® arm of the WHIS made many doctors hesitant to prescribe hormones. They realize it is now necessary to spend more time discussing HRT goals with patients, and to clearly define the reasons for using HRT. Documenting symptoms and linking these symptoms to tested hormone levels assists physicians in supporting the use of hormone replacement in any given patient. Physicians also find that symptoms can be explained in terms of imbalances between the hormone groups.

MENOPAUSE SYMPTOMS

Hormone receptors are present in almost all tissues, so when hormone levels drop, the effects can be felt all over the body. Sex hormone receptors are particularly plentiful in the brain, blood vessels, reproductive organs, urethra (bladder outlet), and bone. Many symptoms are associated with menopause and while some of these symptoms are readily explained by deficiency states or imbalances, others are not. We will briefly describe some of the more common symptoms associated with menopause and, describe how these symptoms relate to hormones.

Anxiety: Anxiety is frequently associated with an excess of estrogen compared to progesterone. Estradiol and progesterone exert opposite effects on brain neurons; progesterone is calming while estradiol is stimulating. Sometimes the progesterone level drops more, relative to estradiol at menopause, leading to a more excitable, anxious state.

Bladder problems: The bladder is rich in estrogen receptors, and declining estrogen levels can cause thinning, or atrophy of the urethra (the passage for urine from the bladder). This may result in frequent bladder and urinary tract infections and/or incontinence. Urinary incontinence is an involuntary leakage of urine that commonly occurs while performing certain activities. Any activity such as laughing or sneezing that increases pressure in the abdominal area may cause the urethral sphincter to open. Small doses of estrogen can often help alleviate this problem.

Bloating: Fluid retention is a frequent cause of bloating. Having too much estrogen or not enough progesterone can cause fluid to accumulate in tissues. Progesterone acts as a natural diuretic and helps to eliminate fluids and reduce the effects of excess estrogen.

Breast tenderness: As you would expect, breast tissue is also rich with hormone receptors. Breast tenderness occurs with a relative excess of estrogens over progesterone. This could be a function of too little progesterone or too much estrogen or both. Actual swelling of the breasts can occur in women who are taking or applying too much progesterone. (The excess progesterone is converted to a metabolite called deoxycorticosterone, which causes the breasts to swell.)

Depression: Deficiencies of estrogens and or androgens can contribute to depression. High evening cortisol levels and excessive use of progesterone are also associated with depression. Women who suffered clinical depression prior to menopause are at greater risk of being depressed in menopause. There are many factors involved in depression, but addressing hormone imbalances may help some women to resolve mood disturbances.

Hot flashes and night sweats: Some women prefer to call them *power surges*, and they can certainly be powerful! A hot flash produces profuse sweating for one to five minutes and can occur as little as a few times each year, or as often as every hour of the day. Approximately three-quarters of women experience hot flashes in menopause. For 15 to 25% of women, hot flashes can be quite debilitating and may even lead to depression and insomnia from night sweats. Hot flashes typically persist for an average of two years, although some women report occurrence of hot flashes for decades after menopause.

Although the precise cause of hot flashes is still unknown, it is clear that they are not strictly a symptom of low estrogen. Women who are prescribed estrogen often get relief from their hot flashes, but we know that women with *high* estrogen levels can also experience hot flashes. In other words, low estrogen levels are not the only explanation for hot flashes. To complicate the issue, women in some cultures do not experience hot flashes at all. Knowing that all women have the same biology, why do some experience hot flashes while others do not?

Body type is one factor that plays a role. Thin women are more likely to experience hot flashes because they have fewer fat cells and therefore less aromatase to convert androgens to estrogens. Women who started menstruating before age 12, women with irregular menstrual cycles and women who entered menopause prior to age 52 all experience more hot flashes.

There are also a number of lifestyle and dietary factors that contribute to the likelihood of experiencing hot flashes. Smoking, consuming alcohol and not having completed high school are all correlated with increased incidence of hot flashes. Diabetes is associated with hot flashes and some women experience hot flashes when sugar is consumed. Stress is also a major factor. Many women do not experience hot flashes until they are hit with a major stressor. Populations that consume a lot of phytoestrogens such as soy foods are less likely to experience hot flashes. Cultural factors may also play a role in hot flashes. Western societies have a generally negative view of the aging process often seeing it as a decline in usefulness, which in turn may lead some women to experience more unpleasant symptoms.

Irritability: Irritability can arise from a number of different hormone issues. Excess estrogen relative to progesterone is a common hormone imbalance that often results in increased irritability. A lack of androgens can also be a factor in irritability, as can an excess of the stress hormone cortisol. If irritability is the predominant symptom, it would be wise to do hormone testing to confirm which of the hormones, if any, is responsible for the symptom. Chapter 6 looks at hormone testing in detail.

Poor concentration, foggy thinking: Estradiol is needed for the transport of glucose into the brain, which means that too little estradiol leads to energy-starved brain cells and foggy

73

thinking. Supplementing with too much progesterone can also contribute to foggy thinking. Too much of the stress hormone cortisol can impair memory, as can a lack of testosterone. If 'foggy thinking' is a major symptom, it is advisable to do hormone testing to confirm which of the hormones is responsible.

Skin: Many women complain of a significant loss of skin elasticity with the onset of menopause. Estrogen is known to help keep skin younger looking and more elastic. For some women, this alone is sufficient reason to take estrogens. It's important to remember that estrogens must always be balanced with progesterone and be used in the smallest possible effective dose.

Sleep disturbances: Estrogen deficiencies contribute directly and indirectly to sleep disturbances. Estrogen replacement therapy has been shown to improve sleep in symptomatic menopausal women. Estrogen deficiency also affects sleep indirectly, as night sweats can make it impossible to sleep through the night. Supplementation with progesterone, particularly oral progesterone, can improve sleep quality.

Vaginal dryness: The cause of hot flashes may be elusive, but vaginal dryness is a direct consequence of decreased estrogen. When estrogen levels drop, it takes a few years for the effects to be noticed, but eventually the drop in estrogen leads to dryness and thinning of cells in the vagina and genital area. Low levels of androgens such as testosterone are also a contributing factor in vaginal dryness since androgens are responsible for maintaining tissues in a healthy, built up state.

Weight gain: Weight gain at the waist can be associated with elevated cortisol levels. High levels of this stress hormone can also cause unstable blood sugar levels and sugar cravings. Weight gain at the hips may occur when there is a relative excess of estrogens over progesterone. Excess estrogens can also impair thyroid function, even if thyroid tests are normal, leading to weight gain. Restoring the balance between these hormones may make weight loss easier, but keep in mind that many factors influence weight in menopause.

SYMPTOM PATTERNS

Many symptoms accompany the arrival of menopause, and while individual symptoms give valuable information on the nature of hormone imbalances in the body, so do patterns of symptoms. For some women, the picture is very clear from symptoms alone. For example relative excess of estrogen over progesterone is usually apparent from symptoms alone. In some cases however, the symptom picture is less clear, and hormone testing will be required to confirm the nature of the imbalance. Here are some of the typical symptom patterns associated with menopausal hormones:

Estrogens

The symptoms associated with estrogen imbalance are listed in Table 2. Many doctors and patients get into trouble with excessive estrogen dosing. There is a right amount of hormone for every tissue. If too much hormone is delivered, cells will defend themselves by reducing the number of estrogen receptors. This is called down-regulation. Receptor down-regulation can result in symptoms of estrogen deficiency even when estrogen is being supplemented in ample amounts. The estrogen is there but the cells can't *see* it. The solution is to cut back on estrogens and let the body readjust. On the estrogen excess side, there are several symptoms that can be associated with low thyroid activity. When too much estrogen is present, it interferes with the action of thyroid hormones inside the cell nucleus, even though thyroid hormone levels may be normal.

Estrogens	
Deficiency	**Excess**
Hot flashes	Mood swings
Night sweats	Breast tenderness
Vaginal dryness	Water retention
Foggy thinking	Foggy thinking
Memory lapses	Irritability
Incontinence	Anxiety
Tearfulness	Fibrocystic breasts
Depression	Weight gain - hips
Disturbed sleep	Bleeding changes
Heart palpitations	Headaches
Bone loss	Uterine fibroids
	Cold body temperature
	Fatigue

Table 2

Progesterone

Table 3 shows the symptoms related to progesterone deficiencies and excesses. A careful look at both estrogen and progesterone symptoms shows that the symptoms of too little progesterone are the same as the symptoms of too much estrogen! This is because the two hormones are so closely linked that neither can work properly without the other. A certain amount of progesterone is needed to *turn on* estradiol receptors. Without this permissive amount of progesterone, higher than normal amounts of estrogen would be required to achieve the same effect.

Progesterone	
Deficiency	**Excess**
Mood swings	Drowsiness
Breast tenderness	Breast swelling
Water retention	Nausea
Foggy thinking	Depression
Irritability	Foggy thinking
Anxiety	Oily skin
Fibrocystic breasts	Increased acne
Weight gain – hips	Excess facial hair
Bleeding changes	
Headaches	
Uterine fibroids	
Cold body temperature	
Fatigue	

Table 3

Symptoms of progesterone excess are almost never encountered outside the context of progesterone replacement. Progesterone excess is more common with oral progesterone because the liver converts it to more soluble 'metabolites' that continue to have an effect on progesterone receptors. Progesterone creams avoid this metabolite-forming *first pass* effect by the liver. Some women convert progesterone to testosterone, and can experience symptoms of excess androgens with progesterone supplementation.

Estrogen and Progesterone Balance

It's very important to remember the balance between these two hormones, instead of thinking just in terms of deficiency and excess. For example, a normal or high normal estradiol level, coupled with normal, low normal or low progesterone can result in an estrogen excess pattern. The respective hormone levels don't have to be off the charts high *or* low. Combining hormone test results with an analysis of symptoms can help identify these situations.

Androgens and Androgen Precursors

Before menopause, about half the circulating testosterone comes from DHEA, which is produced by the adrenal glands. Adrenal imbalance or chronic illness can lead to low DHEA, which can contribute to low testosterone. This problem is more acute after menopause or after removal of the ovaries, because the ovaries no longer contribute to testosterone production. Research activity on androgen replacement in women has increased in the past few years, particularly in women who have had their ovaries removed.

Cortisol plays a key role in androgen function. Studies indicate that cortisol and testosterone work on the same genes, but in opposite ways. In other words, a woman with normal testosterone but an elevated cortisol level could show symptoms of low testosterone. This is an example of a functional deficiency. The level of a hormone may be normal, but the system *functions* as if the hormone level was low. This is why it is important to look at a broad range of hormones, in order to uncover the hidden problems.

Androgens	
Deficiency	**Excess**
Depression	Acne
Fatigue	Oily skin
Bone loss	Excess facial/body hair
Vaginal dryness	Weight gain
Decreased sex drive	Insulin resistance
Sleep disturbances	Polycystic ovaries
Decreased muscle mass	Irritability
Incontinence	Loss of scalp hair
Memory lapses	
Muscle aches/stiffness	
Foggy thinking	

Table 4

Cortisol

Very few physicians think about cortisol, except in terms of profound deficiency (Addison's Disease) and profound excess (Cushing's Syndrome). In truth, there is a whole spectrum in between, and hormone balance cannot be achieved unless cortisol issues are properly addressed. It is important to note that cortisol levels rise and fall throughout the day. Cortisol output is highest within the first hour after waking, declines steadily through the day, and reaches a minimum during sleep. This variation of cortisol throughout the day can be readily mapped using saliva hormone testing. Four saliva specimens are collected: morning (within the first hour of waking), before lunch, before supper, and before bedtime and the four hormone levels are graphed.

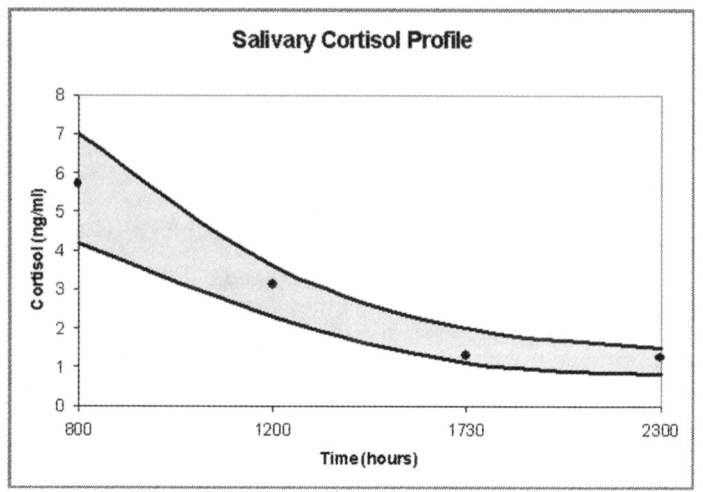

Figure 5

Figure 5 shows how four sample points fit into a normal cortisol range. The shaded area shows the normal daily pattern of cortisol release. Any points falling outside this shaded area might indicate an adrenal problem.

Individuals with a flattened cortisol profile, (no morning rise in cortisol) generally suffer from adrenal fatigue. This often shows up as morning sluggishness, fatigue, low blood sugar, loss of ability to think under pressure, poor exercise tolerance, feeling 'burned out', and/or a sense of being unable to cope with life in general. Another common cortisol profile shows a normal morning surge with higher-than-normal afternoon and evening cortisol levels. Individuals displaying this pattern often have difficulty getting to sleep, feel 'tired but wired' and may have unstable blood sugar. Chronically elevated cortisol can promote bone loss. Chronic mild elevation of cortisol is also associated with hypertension and diabetes and is a fairly common pattern in women diagnosed with breast cancer. A full discussion of all the potential cortisol profiles is beyond the scope of this book, but the book *Adrenal Fatigue: The 21st Century Syndrome* by James Wilson is an excellent resource on this subject. Table 5 has a list of the symptoms associated with cortisol imbalances. Since healthy adrenal glands are essential for postmenopausal production of hormones, signs of cortisol deficiencies or excesses should be promptly and thoroughly investigated.

Cortisol

Deficiency	Excess
Fatigue	Irritable
Allergies	'Tired but wired' feeling
Aching muscles	Weight gain waist
Feeling cold	Loss of muscle mass
Neck stiffness	Bone loss
Increased infections	High blood pressure
Morning sluggishness	Insulin resistance
'Burned out' feeling	Low sex drive
Low sex drive	Impaired memory
Feel unable to cope	'Burned out' feeling
	Loss of scalp hair
	Depression

Table 5

Thyroid Hormone

Functional hypothyroidism is an extremely common problem that probably affects thousands of Canadians. With functional hypothyroidism, thyroid tests are normal, but all the symptoms of low thyroid or hypothyroidism are present. There are many possible contributing factors to functional hypothyroidism including: deficiencies of nutrients like selenium and zinc, too much estrogen, too little progesterone, and too much or too little cortisol. The following is a typical example of functional hypothyroidism: a 35-year-old woman has her uterus and ovaries removed, and is put on oral estrogen replacement therapy. She is not given progesterone because her doctor says she doesn't need it since her uterus is gone! Months later she has gained 30 pounds, is tired all the time, feels like she can never get warm, and her hair is starting to thin. Thyroid tests are normal and her doctor says there's nothing he can do for her. This woman is experiencing a functional thyroid deficiency due to the effect of unopposed estrogen (estrogen not balanced by progesterone). The solution to her problem is simple: give her progesterone! She may not have her uterus, but she still has the rest of her body, and *all* estrogen-sensitive tissues are used to a balance between estrogens and progesterone.

These are but a few examples of the complex array of symptoms associated with hormone imbalances. Sometimes the hormone imbalances can cause a particular condition to develop, as in the cases of functional hypothyroidism and functional androgen deficiency. Occasionally, a collection of symptoms points to the start of a chronic illness or disease. There are several diseases of concern in menopausal women, and what follows is a discussion of the role of hormones in these diseases.

DISEASES

Bone Loss (Osteoporosis) or thinning of the bones, is a major concern in postmenopausal women. Hip fractures are a frequent cause of hospitalization in elderly women and are associated with shortened life expectancy. As with hot flashes, there are a number of lifestyle and physiological factors that contribute to bone loss. Risk factors include: being small-boned, being a smoker, having a low calcium intake, doing little or no weight bearing exercise, being fair skinned, and having high caffeine intake.

Hormones also play a significant role in the development of osteoporosis, as hormone receptors are abundant in bone. Deficiencies in estrogen and testosterone (an androgen) as well as an excess of cortisol can all contribute to significant bone loss. For women who have experienced significant bone loss, supplementation with estrogen and/or testosterone combined with stress reduction strategies may be indicated. The choice of hormone(s) should be made based on the symptom inventory and confirmatory hormone testing. The role of progesterone in bone is still being investigated, but so far the evidence suggests that progesterone alone does not increase bone density. However, progesterone may assist the action of other bone-building hormones (e.g. estradiol).

Breast Cancer is a major concern for women of all ages. Estrogens may act as initiators of cancer or as promoters of cancer cell growth. As mentioned previously, there are concerns about excess estrogen metabolites such as estrone sulphate and 4-hydroxyestrone. However, not all hormones are equivalent when it comes to breast cancer risk. Estriol, the weakest estrogen, may have a protective effect against breast cancer. Progesterone may also reduce the risk of developing breast cancer via its balancing effects on estrogen. This is in contrast to the effects of the synthetic progestin MPA (Provera®), which has been shown to *increase* breast cancer risk.

Breast cancer is an area where having the right hormone key for the receptor lock is critical. A British study showed that women with breast cancer whose progesterone level at the time of surgery was above a certain level had significantly improved chances of survival. Progesterone is needed to regulate a class of enzymes known as metalloproteinases. Cancer cells use these enzymes to invade tissue and develop their blood supply. The ability of progesterone to regulate metalloproteinases may mean that progesterone can be protective against cancers in general. Women looking for more information on the role hormones play in breast cancer should read Dr. John Lee and Dr. David Zava's book *What Your Doctor May Not Tell You About Breast Cancer,* in which they discuss the role that hormone balance plays in breast cancer, and what women can do to assess and modify their breast cancer risk.

Heart Disease is significantly more prevalent in post-menopausal women. No one is sure exactly why this is the case. It is likely a combination of lower hormone levels, cumulative stress, lifestyle and nutritional issues. Estrogen is essential for healthy functioning of blood vessels and it has been theorized that the drop in estrogen at menopause is partially responsible for the increased risk of heart disease. Various studies, and most notably, the WHIS, have indicated that higher dose oral estrogens and synthetic progestins are not good for the heart, but the studies looking at the effect of bio-identical hormones on tissue supports what we have known all along: human hormones delivered in ways the body is familiar with, are not the enemy of human beings!

Polycystic Ovary Disease (PCOD) is a collection of symptoms that correlate with high androgen levels. Women with PCOD may experience irregular or absent periods as well as the symptoms of androgen excess such as excess facial and body hair. Many women with PCOD also struggle with obesity and insulin resistance.

SUMMARY

Symptoms are an excellent way to begin to assess hormonal status, but the assessment shouldn't stop there. There are many ways in which hormones silently interact, and these can only be uncovered by testing. Also, hormone overdoses can be silent, with the accumulation of potentially harmful metabolites that may not cause symptoms but can increase the risk of long-term health problems. Hormone testing can help identify potential hormone overdoses, and clarify confusing symptom patterns. In the wake of the Women's Health Initiative Study, there is a need to approach hormone replacement methodically and document the rationale for its use. Collecting and analyzing information on symptoms is simply good medical practice. Putting the symptoms together with test results is a great strategy for hitting the hormone replacement target.

CHAPTER SIX

STEP 2
Uncovering Imbalances with Hormone Testing

Step 1 outlined the importance of looking at symptoms to determine whether a hormone imbalance is present. The second step on the path to restoring hormone balance involves confirmation of imbalances through testing. In this chapter, we'll discuss the options available for hormone testing, and how they can help uncover hormone imbalances.

HORMONE TESTING

Laboratory Medicine has really only evolved in the last 50 or 60 years, with major advances occurring in the last 30 years. Prior to this, lab tests were simple procedures done by the physicians themselves, in their offices. In those days there was no separation of the patient and the laboratory; the physician *was* the laboratory, and he knew the patient intimately and was immediately able to connect the lab test result to the patient's problem. Now of course, the situation in clinical chemistry has changed. The laboratory's only role for many patients is simply to provide numbers, and do it accurately and efficiently.

87

Consider what happens when lab tests are done in isolation from the patients. Typically, normal ranges are developed by testing large numbers of people. The spread of the results is analyzed and the normal ranges are derived on a statistical basis. This approach often doesn't take individual variation into account. For some people, a result in the middle of the range is low, or a result at the low end of the range is normal. It depends on the individual's particular hormone needs, and on the balance of many factors: other hormones, enzymes, and nutritional co-factors.

In the case of hormone testing, this is what we want to know: what does this *number* mean for a given patient? The physician ordering the test can certainly put everything together once he or she has the result, by looking back over the chart and consulting notes regarding symptoms, use of supplements and other medical issues. But most physicians don't have the time to do this kind of in-depth analysis. This is where the laboratory can step in and fill the breach by collecting clinical information with each sample and interpreting the test results in the context of the patient's symptoms. As was mentioned last chapter, this approach is particularly relevant given the results of the Women's Health Initiative (see Introduction). Documentation and a reasoned approach to HRT are mandatory now for any physician contemplating hormone replacement therapy.

A discussion of the success of this holistic approach to laboratory medicine, which considers symptoms along with hormone levels, comes later. First, here's a comparison of the major testing modalities: blood, urine and saliva, from the standpoint of relevance, convenience and other practical considerations.

HORMONE TRANSPORT

Hormone testing is complicated business. The structures of the various hormones are similar, and this can make it hard to tell one hormone from another. The hormones travel through the blood in at least three different forms: free, protein-bound, and red blood cell-bound. The amounts of some of the forms are quite tiny, measured in trillionths of grams per specimen. Researchers don't fully understand the roles of these different forms and each type of lab test measures a different combination of these forms. No wonder people are confused about lab testing, and this includes laboratorians!

Actually, hormone transportation can be broken down into fairly simple terms. Steroid hormones are oily substances, and the *free* steroids are like individual *droplets* of oil suspended in the watery matrix of the blood. Also floating in the blood are spongy *blobs* that can soak up many droplets of oil. These blobs are proteins such as albumin and sex hormone binding globulin. Finally, there are the *supertankers*, or red blood cells, which can carry a big load of oil on their spongy surfaces, or stored in their hulls (cell membranes).

For a long time, most researchers believed that only the free hormone form (droplets) was available to act on tissues (bioavailable). We have come to realize however, that all forms are bioavailable, depending on the target tissue we are talking about, and depending on whether the hormones are produced naturally or are being supplemented. Different tests look at different forms of hormones (free, protein bound or red blood cell bound). As a consequence, the answers don't always come out the same when we compare results using different methods.

TEST MODALITIES
Blood

Blood testing can be divided into two categories: serum testing and whole blood. Serum testing involves a trip to the lab and a needle poke in the arm. A tube of blood is drawn, and the watery yellow serum is separated out and sent to the lab for analysis. Whole blood testing can be done at home using a lancet, getting a drop of blood from the fingertip similar to the way blood glucose testing is done for diabetes. The whole blood spot is allowed to dry on a piece of filter paper, and mailed back to the lab.

Serum testing primarily measures total hormone: the *blobby* protein-bound form plus the *droplet* free form. Free *unbound* hormone can be measured separately but this test is only available through specialized laboratories in the United States. Depending on how a dried blood spot is processed, all the hormone components can be measured. Currently however, only protein-bound hormones are measured in blood spot, the same as for serum. Blood spot testing of hormones has only recently become available in the U.S. and is not yet available in Canada.

All the common hormones can be measured in serum although estrogens are limited: estrone sulphate is not available and the estriol test only measures the higher levels seen in pregnant women. A limited range of hormones is currently available for blood spot testing, again, due to the newness of this testing method.

Whole blood spot testing is convenient since it can be done at home, and multiple samples can be taken in a given day if necessary. Conversely, serum testing involves a trip to a laboratory to have blood drawn and is therefore less convenient, especially since it is best to test some hormones within an hour of waking (e.g. cortisol). Nevertheless, serum testing is the most widely used testing, in part by default. Many physicians don't realize these other tests exist! Also, serum testing is paid for by government-funded health insurance plans, at least for the time being. In this climate of health care cost-cutting, it is quite likely that serum hormone testing will come under scrutiny eventually, since some people consider testing hormones medically unnecessary!

One final point: with serum hormone tests you just get the number, since the lab doesn't get any information about you except your name, sex and date of birth.

Urine

Urine has been used very successfully for decades to assess steroid hormones. Typically, the measurements are made on a small portion of all the urine collected in a 24-hour period, and this is both a strength and weakness. Twenty-four hour collection smoothes out the fluctuations in

91

hormone production and gives a good indicator of average daily production, but 24-hour collection is inconvenient for the patient.

For the most part, hormones that appear in urine have been conjugated or processed by the liver to make them more soluble. The hormones bound to carrier proteins and red blood cells, as well as the free hormones, are not conjugated. So urine testing is misleading because we are looking at hormone the body is trying to get rid of, not the hormone that is actually getting into tissue. Nevertheless, urinary hormone levels reflect the body's total output of a given hormone, and a wide range of hormones can be measured. Urine testing also differentiates between similar metabolites whereas blood tests can lump two, three or twenty similar hormone metabolites together and report one number, which is higher than it should be.

Currently, cortisol is the only hormone test commonly available in urine and covered by government health insurance. Several specialized laboratories in the U.S. offer comprehensive panels in urine, but as with serum tests, the laboratory receives limited patient information. The lack of a symptom assessment with the test results means that the information may be of limited value.

Saliva

Researchers began studying saliva as a vehicle to test hormones more than 20 years ago, but this form of testing for steroid hormones is just now reaching wide acceptance. For drugs of abuse, saliva has surpassed urine as the sample type of choice.

Saliva testing has many advantages. Samples can be taken at home; multiple samples can be acquired painlessly throughout the day, and samples can be mailed in to the lab. A wider range of hormones is available in saliva than in blood or serum. Although saliva testing is generally not covered by government insurance plans, private insurance plans often cover it.

In order to understand the critical difference between saliva tests and blood tests, it's necessary to understand how hormones get into saliva. The hormones measured in saliva have to escape the blood, pass through the capillary walls and make their way to the cell membranes of the cells lining the saliva duct. Then a small amount of hormone will leave the cell membranes and go into the saliva being formed in the duct. This means saliva testing measures hormone that has been delivered to tissues: the bioavailable hormone. Recall that hormones are distributed in three main forms in the blood, and that all 3 forms are available to tissues. Saliva appears to be sensitive to *all three* forms of hormone, and unlike urine and blood tests, it can detect hormone carried on red blood cell *supertankers*. This is particularly important when we are trying to do hormone tests on people using hormone creams.

Skin delivery of hormones enriches the hormone content of the red blood cells to some degree. These cells then travel quickly (within seconds) to other parts of the body and unload their hormones. This takes place so fast that the watery part of the blood can't keep up. When hormones are delivered through the skin, large increases in saliva hormone levels occur, but the corresponding changes in blood levels are small. Many physicians have used this apparent discrepancy to discount the value of both saliva testing and transdermal hormone delivery. In Chapter Four however, we discussed the evidence showing that hormones delivered via skin get to the desired tissues. Saliva is currently the only test method available that can detect hormone on red blood cells, which is how hormones appear to be transported when delivered through the skin. Many practitioners who have used all three types of testing (blood, urine and saliva) state that saliva testing tends to correlate better to the clinical picture. This is consistent with the idea that a saliva level is really a salivary tissue level. Chapter Four also cited an experiment in which rats were given progesterone cream and the levels of progesterone in various tissues were measured. There was twice as much progesterone in salivary tissue as in blood, and 8 times as much progesterone in uterine tissue compared to blood. This supports the notion that saliva levels better reflect levels in other body tissues, although more research in this area needs to be done. Simply put, saliva hormone levels are an excellent measure of tissue levels of hormone because hormones have to pass through tissue to get into saliva.

The Best Test

A question often posed by physicians and patients who are new to bio-identical hormone replacement is, what is the best test? The honest answer is that there is no best test. No test can tell a practitioner what specific hormone dose to start a patient with, or what adjustment to make to an existing dose. The practitioner must make these decisions based on his or her experience and the patient's symptoms. However, tests are extremely useful for identifying hormone imbalance, and for alerting practitioners to the need for a dosage adjustment. Throwing hormones at a problem before accurately identifying the problem is a risky way to practice. Hormone testing helps identify the problems.

There is a wonderfully complex interplay between hormones at the level of DNA in the nucleus of every cell. When we test, we are looking at the system from much further away. Looking at hormones in blood is like Nancy Drew hiding behind a bush and peering at a pile of packages stacked outside a house. She doesn't know if the packages will go into the house, or what will be done with them if they wind up inside. With hormones in urine, it's like Nancy is looking through the trash, again trying to figure out what's going on inside the house. With saliva testing, Nancy has sneaked up to the window, but she can still only see into one room, so the view isn't quite perfect.

A better view can be obtained by gathering clinical information with each specimen. This includes age, height, weight, details on menstrual status, gynaecological surgical history, supplemental hormones, nutritionals and pharmaceuticals, and a detailed inventory of hormone-related symptoms. Laboratories gathering comprehensive clinical information (see Resources) use this information to improve the view offered by hormone testing. The test report provides a link between hormone levels and the symptom profile and suggestions for restoring the balance of hormones can be made. Measuring a broad array of hormones often yields insight into the cause of symptoms, and shows how hormones can affect one another via their complex interactions. Unfortunately, few labs take the time to gather clinical information to assist in the interpretation of hormone test results.

Saliva testing probably gives the best view of hormone actions, but like Nancy Drew, practitioners should look at the situation from many different angles, gather as many clues as possible, and integrate the information in a way that benefits the patient. It's important that practitioners just *start* to do hormone testing of some kind, to make their approach to hormone replacement as objective as possible. Practitioners need to become students of the art of hormone testing and HRT. The laboratory's job is to assist practitioners with their learning, and provide a service, rather than simply giving numbers. In the words of a physician who had her own saliva test done by a lab that collects clinical information; "the report was exactly what I had predicted before I did the test and was reassuring to me that I am not crazy... The report format is very useful and I will certainly recommend doing the test to other friends and patients". Clearly, practitioners and laboratories can work together to give women the information they need to solve their hormone problems.

CHAPTER SEVEN

STEP 3
Restoring Hormone Balance

A thorough symptom assessment along with hormone testing gives a useful, though somewhat incomplete, picture of what the hormones are doing in the tissues. Restoring hormone balance isn't always a simple process of supplementing one hormone or another. Sometimes hormone imbalances can be best addressed by making better lifestyle and dietary choices. For some women, restoring the balance of hormones simply involves switching from non-human/synthetic hormones to natural/bio-identical hormones. Sometimes hormone imbalances can lead to, or are signs of, other health problems. For example, polycystic ovary disease and insulin resistance can be associated with specific hormone imbalances. Restoring hormone balance is often complex, but can significantly improve the health of the women who achieve it.

It's impossible to describe all the possible combinations of hormone imbalances, but the following sample cases illustrate some common patterns that emerge from Symptom Analysis and Hormone Testing.

TINA

Tina is a 58 year old woman who had a hysterectomy in her 40's and has been on Premarin® ever since. She was told she didn't need progesterone since she her uterus had been removed. After the result of the WHIS were announced, Tina stopped her Premarin® cold turkey, with unfortunate consequences. She began having hot flashes again, became mildly depressed, and felt 'foggy' in her thinking.

Saliva testing showed Tina's estradiol level was very low as was her testosterone. Her family doctor recommended commercial estradiol gel, Estrogel®, at a dose of 2 pumps per day. Two pumps a day delivers 1.5 mg of estradiol, nearly the same dose as would be given orally. Recall that only 10% of oral estradiol stays as estradiol; with the rest being broken down into metabolites by the liver. Estradiol delivered through skin goes to tissues as estradiol before going to the liver. Luckily, Tina spoke to someone knowledgeable in hormone delivery and opted to only apply ¼ pump of Estrogel® daily, or 0.188mg. She also started on 20mg of progesterone cream once daily.

Tina's symptoms immediately improved. A repeat saliva hormone test showed her estradiol was still twice normal, and she was advised to cut her Estrogel® dose even further. She is scheduled for a retest after her dose is stabilized. Testosterone supplementation may be an option once estradiol and progesterone are in balance.

SALLY

History

Sally Smith is a very fit, lean, 55 year-old businesswoman trying to *do* menopause naturally. Her periods stopped two years ago, but she still suffers from hot flashes, memory lapses, vaginal dryness, foggy thinking, low sex drive, bladder problems *and* disturbed sleep! Sally has a very stressful job. There is no family history of breast cancer, heart disease or osteoporosis. She has not had a bone density scan.

Symptom Analysis

Sally's symptoms are suggestive of low estrogen (hot flashes, vaginal dryness, foggy thinking) and testosterone levels (low sex drive, fatigue, vaginal dryness, urinary incontinence).

Saliva Hormone Test Results

Estradiol: <1.5 pg/ml   (low)

Progesterone: 30 pg/ml   (normal for menopause)

Testosterone: 15 pg/ml   (low normal)

Cortisol AM: 10 ng/ml   (high)

DHEAS: 4.5 ng/ml   (low normal)

Saliva Test Interpretation

Low estradiol contributes to symptoms of estrogen deficiency including vaginal dryness, memory lapses, hot flashes and incontinence. Progesterone is necessary for optimal functioning of estradiol as well as thyroid hormones. Supplementation with bio-identical progesterone alone may be helpful in symptom relief. For example, a one-year trial of progesterone cream demonstrated efficacy compared to placebo, for the control of vasomotor symptoms (Leonetti HB, Longo S, Anasti JN. *Transdermal progesterone cream for vasomotor symptoms and postmenopausal bone loss.* Obstet Gynecol. 1999 Aug;94(2):225-228). After menopause, the supply of testosterone comes from DHEA of adrenal origin, hence the low normal testosterone is consistent with low normal DHEAS. Supplementation with bio-identical testosterone may be worth exploring to address issues of decrease libido and incontinence. Elevated morning cortisol often reflects stress and in general opposes the action of the other hormones. Elevated cortisol, low estradiol and low testosterone put this individual at risk for osteoporosis; consideration should be given to having a bone density scan.

Recommendations for Sally

Testing confirmed suspicions about low estrogen and testosterone levels, and also revealed an adrenal issue; low DHEAS coupled with high cortisol. A physician experienced in BHRT might do the following, after receiving this report:

- Counsel Sally on reducing stress.
- Suggest supplements to support adrenal function or refer Sally to a naturopath.
- Obtain a bone density scan-to use as a baseline and to monitor therapy
- Suggest a mammogram and/or breast thermal imaging (can be used as a baseline to monitor long term effect of estrogen supplementation on breast density and thermal properties of breasts)
- Transdermal estrogen 25 days/month (slow release patch or compounded estrogen skin cream). May need to use a higher starting dose, and reduce after a month or so.

- Transdermal progesterone 25 days/month commencing 2 weeks after starting estrogen. This gives the estrogen time to *prime* the body and increase the production of progesterone receptors.
- Repeat saliva estradiol and progesterone tests after 2 months on both hormones to make sure the estrogen dose is not too high and to confirm delivery of progesterone to tissue.
- Assess need for testosterone after 3 months of other therapies. Stress reduction alone may improve libido. Consider starting bio-identical testosterone cream (0.5-1.0 mg/daily) if no improvement.
- See patient at 2-month intervals for the rest of the first year.
- Repeat bone density, breast imaging and saliva tests at 1 year.

ALEXANDRA

History

Alexandra is a slightly overweight 47 year-old woman who is experiencing a number of unpleasant symptoms. Alexandra complains of irritability, foggy thinking, mood swings, anxiety, bloating and headaches. She has numerous small fibrous cysts or lumps in her breast. She's starting to gain weight around the hips, and has noticed that her periods are quite irregular and she's bleeding heavily. Her doctor also recently told her she has uterine fibroids or small *knots* in the muscle of the uterus that can cause heavier, crampier periods. As discussed in Chapter 5, Alexandra's symptoms are consistent with estrogen excess, also called estrogen dominance.

Saliva Test Results

Estradiol	5 pg/ml	(high normal)
Progesterone	85 pg/ml	(low normal for luteal phase)
Testosterone	40 pg/ml	(high)

Saliva Test Interpretation

Both estradiol and progesterone are within normal limits, however symptoms of fibrocystic breasts, fibroids, weight gain and headaches are consistent with a relative excess of estradiol (not enough progesterone to balance estradiol). Supplementation with bio-identical progesterone during the luteal phase might be beneficial. There is an association between elevated testosterone and insulin resistance; insulin resistance in turn is associated with an increased risk of heart disease and diabetes. Regular exercise including weight training and elimination of refined carbohydrates from the diet might be helpful. Reduced estrogen exposure through avoidance of commercially raised beef and poultry might be a prudent strategy.

Recommendations for Alexandra

It is clear from Alexandra's symptoms and saliva hormone results that some form of hormone intervention is necessary. Part of her problem arises from the fact that her periods are irregular and she is failing to ovulate in some cycles. When ovulation doesn't occur, progesterone isn't produced and estrogen dominance is the result. Because her symptoms result from estrogen excess, and because she is still menstruating, Alexandra doesn't need more estrogen. Symptom relief will come from supplementation with progesterone (e.g. progesterone cream, 15-30 mg/day, 2 or 3 weeks/month). Progesterone acts as a natural diuretic and may assist Alexandra in shedding excess pounds caused by fluid retention. Estrogen dominance is also associated with weight gain at the hips, so giving progesterone may help Alexandra shave off a few centimeters from her hips. Weight loss will also help decrease the amount of estrogen Alexandra produces via the aromatase enzyme in the fat cells. Most women find progesterone has a calming effect, so Alexandra should notice reduced anxiety and irritability once she starts using progesterone. Small uterine fibroids and fibrocystic breasts also respond well to progesterone. The possibility of insulin resistance is another concern raised by Alexandra's test results. With insulin resistance, the body begins to *resist* the effects of insulin and has to produce more insulin to control blood glucose levels. Insulin resistance is a warning that full-blown diabetes may not be far away. It is directly linked to consumption of too much refined sugar and white flour. Muscle is very glucose-hungry so weight training will help Alexandra absorb glucose from her blood more readily, and reduce her insulin output.

JEAN
History

Jean is a 42 year-old woman who had a hysterectomy last year due to uterine fibroids. She still has her ovaries. She began to experience hot flashes several months after her surgery, told her doctor about it and was informed this was impossible because she still had her ovaries. She is fatigued, her allergies have gotten worse, and she has all the same symptoms as Sally plus she's suffering from depression.

103

She feels cold all the time and can't seem to get going in the mornings. Her doctor recently started her on an antidepressant.

Symptom Analysis

Jean's symptoms are suggestive of low estradiol (hot flashes, depression), low testosterone (fatigue, decreased libido) low cortisol (fatigue, worsening allergies, can't get started in mornings) and hypothyroidism (fatigue and feeling cold).

Saliva Hormone Test Results

Estradiol: 1.5 pg/ml   (low)
Progesterone: 20 pg/ml   (low)
Testosterone: 17 pg/ml   (low normal)
Cortisol AM: 2.5 ng/ml   (low)
DHEA-S: 6 ng/ml   (normal)

Saliva Test Interpretation

Low estradiol, progesterone and testosterone are suggestive of ovarian failure, which is common after hysterectomy. These deficiencies may contribute to symptoms of estrogen deficiency including vaginal dryness, memory lapses, hot flashes and incontinence. Low bioavailable testosterone may be associated with decreased sex drive, depressed mood, decreased enjoyment of life and vaginal dryness. In a recent study by Orozco, salivary testosterone also correlated to bone density (Orozco P et al. Eur J Epidemiol 2000;16-907-912.) Fatigue and worsening allergies may be consistent with failure to elevate morning cortisol. Impaired adrenal function is common after stressors such as surgery. Cortisol is necessary for proper action of thyroid hormones and low cortisol can present with symptoms of hypothyroidism despite normal thyroid tests.

Recommendations for Jean

This case nicely illustrates the complex interplay between hormones and symptoms and is typical of the experience of many women. Even though Jean has her ovaries, they are intended to work in concert with the uterus. Removal of the uterus often triggers ovarian failure, although this effect is not *officially* recognized. Nevertheless, Jean now has the hormone profile of a postmenopausal woman and is at risk for osteoporosis. Furthermore, the stress of surgery may have impaired her adrenal function, which can lead to symptoms of hypothyroidism. Jean needs a two-pronged intervention directed towards supporting her adrenal function and supplementing the ovarian hormones progesterone and estradiol. Low testosterone is also an issue, but her symptoms may improve if her adrenal function (indicated by cortisol levels) is restored to normal. She will have to reassess her symptoms and hormone levels in a few months. If her estradiol, progesterone and testosterone levels have not increased and she is still symptomatic, dosage adjustments may be required. She may also need to consider supplementing with testosterone. Jean also needs to have a bone density scan done. Restoring balance for Jean's hormones may make antidepressant therapy unnecessary.

THERESA
History
Theresa is 45, has regular periods but complains of low sex drive, depression and fatigue since her divorce six months ago. She is a vegetarian.

Symptom Analysis
Theresa's symptoms are not specific to any particular pattern of hormone imbalance.

Saliva Hormone Test Results
Estradiol: 3.7 pg/ml   (normal)
Progesterone: 120 pg/ml   (normal Day 19 luteal phase)
Testosterone: 30 pg/ml   (normal)
Cortisol AM: 15 ng/ml   (high)
DHEAS: 10 ng/ml   (normal)

Saliva Test Interpretation
Morning cortisol is high, and this is often seen in the setting of chronic stress. Cortisol may interfere with the action of other hormones such as testosterone, leading to functional deficiency symptoms.

Recommendations for Theresa
Theresa's main problems appear to be stress and depression. Her high cortisol level is not necessarily linked to depression, but rather the high cortisol is a sign of ongoing stress co-existent with depression. She has an increased risk of developing depression because of her vegetarian diet. Some vegetarians don't consume enough protein. Protein is broken down to amino acids, which are the building blocks for neurotransmitters. Neurotransmitters like serotonin and

norepinephrine are chemical messengers that the brain neurons use to talk to one other. Neurotransmitter deficiencies can lead to depression and anxiety, as well as obesity. Theresa might want to consider having the urinary levels of her neurotransmitters measured, as this testing can help guide supplementation with specific amino acids intended to increase neurotransmitter levels naturally.

MARTHA

History

Martha is 52, and is about 35 pounds overweight. She hasn't had a period in two years, and didn't experience any hot flashes or other obvious menopause symptoms. She has a history of fibrocystic breasts and her mother had uterine cancer. She eats a lot of commercially raised chicken and turkey, as well as some red meat. Martha complains of fatigue, constipation, weight gain and thinning hair.

Symptom Analysis

Martha's symptoms (fatigue, weight gain etc.) are suggestive of hypothyroidism.

Saliva Hormone Test Results

Estradiol: 8 pg/ml   (high)

Progesterone: 25 pg/ml   (low)

Testosterone: 22 pg/ml   (normal)

Cortisol AM: 5.3 ng/ml   (normal)

DHEAS: 4.5 ng/ml   (normal)

Saliva Test Interpretation

Estradiol is higher than expected for a postmenopausal woman who is not replacing estrogens. There is a relative excess of estradiol compared to progesterone. Typical symptoms would include breast tenderness, fluid retention, headaches, and irritability. In this case, the excess of estrogens may instead be acting to impair thyroid function. Symptoms of hypothyroidism include fatigue, feeling cold all the time, thinning hair and constipation. Supplementation with bio-identical progesterone may help to balance estradiol and improve thyroid function. At the same time, increased fiber intake, weight loss and avoidance of commercially raised meat and poultry will help to reduce her estrogen burden.

Recommendations

Martha did well through menopause because she still makes ample estrogens from the aromatase in her body fat, and possibly because she is being exposed to estrogens in her diet. (Commercially raised cattle and poultry are fed estrogens to bring them to market weight faster.) The excess of estrogens over progesterone has probably given Martha a functional thyroid deficiency, which can be managed by giving Martha progesterone. Testing was very beneficial in this case because Martha's symptoms would not ordinarily have been associated with a sex hormone imbalance. Progesterone should help relieve the symptoms of hypothyroidism and help Martha reduce her risk of developing uterine cancer.

DAGNY

History

Dagny is 52 years old and has been on progesterone skin cream, 60 mg/day for two months. Initially she had good relief from her hot flushes and night sweats, and an increase in sex drive, but lately, her hot flushes have started to return.

Symptom Analysis

Dagny's symptoms suggest estrogen deficiency.

Saliva Hormone Test Results

Estradiol: 3.5 pg/ml   (normal)

Progesterone: 50,000 pg/ml   (high)

Saliva Test Interpretation

Estradiol is normal; progesterone is higher than expected for topical use of progesterone.

Recommendations for Dagny

As we pointed out earlier, proper function of any hormone depends on having the right balance. Here, the salivary progesterone level is higher than normally observed and symptoms of estrogen deficiency have re-occurred. When progesterone is in excess over estradiol, this shuts down, or down-regulates the estradiol receptors. Once again, we have a functional deficiency, where the estradiol level is normal, but the message doesn't get through. It turns out Dagny had used her cream every day for two months where she should have been taking a break for at least 5 days each month. She stopped her cream for 10 days, and then restarted at half her dose, being sure to take a short break each month. She is now into her sixth month on the cream and doing fine.

MAKING THE SWITCH FROM PREMARIN® AND PROVERA® TO BHRT

As discussed early in the book, the results of the Women's Health Initiative have caused concern for women using the combination of conjugated equine estrogens and MPA. Many women and their physicians have wisely made the decision, without even looking at symptoms or hormone tests, to switch to more natural forms of hormones. Unfortunately, there is no information available to women to assist them in making this switch, so we offer the following example to illustrate how this transition might best be managed.

SASHA

History

Sasha is 63 years old and has been on Premarin® and Provera® (MPA-medroxyprogesterone acetate) for 11 years. She has decided she wants to switch to bio-identical hormone therapy and isn't sure how to proceed. She feels fine apart from some occasional breast tenderness and fluid retention. Her sex drive is normal. She still has her uterus and ovaries.

Symptom Analysis

Sasha's symptoms (breast tenderness, fluid retention) suggest that she may have an excess of estrogen relative to progesterone.

Saliva Hormone Test Results

Estradiol: 15 pg/ml   (high)
Progesterone: 20 pg/ml   (low)

Testosterone: 23 pg/ml (normal)

Cortisol AM: 6 ng/ml (normal)

DHEAS: 5 ng/ml (normal)

Saliva Test Interpretation

Estradiol is higher than expected for a woman using estrogen. Provera® does not have the same molecular structure as progesterone, and does not register as progesterone in this assay. There are symptoms of estrogen dominance. Bio-identical progesterone might be an option to consider in place of Provera®.

Recommendations for Sasha

Sasha has done reasonably well on her current regimen, although she has some symptoms of estrogen dominance. If she wants to switch to bio-identical hormones, it will require time and patience on her part. Her saliva level indicates that she is carrying too much estradiol and this, coupled with the use of Provera®, has caused estrogen dominant symptoms. The first step is to stop Provera® and start bio-identical progesterone, either cream or oral, 25 days/month. At the same time, Sasha can start reducing her dose of oral estrogen. This can be accomplished by taking a pill every other day, or by halving the dose and taking it every day. If after 2 to 4 weeks Sasha is still free of estrogen deficiency symptoms, she can halve her Premarin® dose again. If Sasha continues to be symptom-free, she can keep lowering her estrogen until she is off it completely. She might do just fine with progesterone alone, 25 days a month. If she decides to go with progesterone alone, Sasha will need to have her bone density monitored on a regular basis.

Many women do run into trouble though, while cutting down on their Premarin® dose. The liver gets used to processing oral estrogen, and produces a certain pattern of enzymes to deal with it. If oral estrogen is stopped, the liver needs time and help to revert back to normal. This manifests itself as an estrogen deficiency, with such symptoms as foggy thinking, hot flashes, and depression. There are several options at this point. Using various natural treatments including herbs, vitamins, and minerals, the liver can learn to adapt to life without oral estrogen. Most naturopathic physicians are skilled in this area.

Another option is to deliver a small amount of estradiol through the skin, enough to keep the symptoms at bay, while continuing to reduce the oral estrogen dose. Once the oral estrogen is stopped, then the transdermal dose can be titrated downward or upward according to symptoms and/or test results.

Making the switch from Premarin® and Provera® to BHRT requires patience, but the long-term benefits to health are well worth the effort. The combination of conjugated equine estrogens and MPA is clearly associated with increased risks of both heart disease and breast cancer. Potentially safer alternatives exist, and can be explored with a little patience.

SUMMARY

Through these various examples, we hope we have been able to illustrate how consideration of symptoms together with hormone testing (in this case salivary hormone testing) can help solve a wide range of health problems. Of course there are situations where the test results don't match the clinical situation, and this simply indicates that there are other factors at play. In Theresa's case, for example, we needed to consider other problems such as inadequate protein intake leading to neurotransmitter deficiencies.

These 3 Simple Steps: Symptom Assessment, Hormone Testing and Restoring the Balance form the basis for an excellent opening dialogue between a woman and her physician. The concerns about hormone replacement have made physicians much more cautious about starting or even continuing hormone replacement therapy. Measuring hormone levels and documenting information on symptoms is simply good medical practice. This book offers women and their physicians a sensible approach to hormone replacement therapy, in this time of uncertainty.

CHAPTER EIGHT

A Call to Action

We wrote this book because women deserve to know the truth about hormones. Women need to know how to find out if they have a hormone imbalance, and what their hormone replacement options are if they have an imbalance. The pharmaceutical companies have their tentacles firmly embedded in medical schools, and physicians feel this influence throughout their careers. This isn't all bad. There are many life-saving drugs on the market. But it seems likely that the interests of women have been subverted by the profit motive when it comes to hormone replacement. The large pharmaceutical companies fund the big studies, and the common-sense bio-identical approaches are left in the lurch when it comes time to design these big trials.

There are rays of hope coming through the clouds. Consider the words of a Canadian family physician that recently appeared in The Medical Post; "So...to the academics and funders of academics: Please, let's have the evidence we need! Let's do well-constructed studies asking useful questions and measuring the outcomes of interest to the subjects concerned - and let's be sure to study the human hormones. Furthermore, until we have done randomized controlled trials with human hormones, *let's not*

114

confuse absence of evidence with evidence of absence"(emphasis ours). In other words, just because the evidence in favour of BHRT is incomplete, let's not assume there is no evidence!

It's your body, and you have the right to access human hormone therapies based on principles of human physiology. We get calls from frustrated women every day: women whose physicians refuse to prescribe bio-identical hormones. We encourage you to go forward and continue to educate yourself and your physician about hormones and hormone balance.

We believe there are many doctors out there who are willing to listen, willing to change, and are willing to proceed in the face of uncertainty, *if* they can be presented with some plain speech about HRT.

The Society of Obstetricians and Gynecologists of Canada (SOGC) and the Canadian Pharmacists Association (CPhA) published a booklet called "Tearing Down The Myths: Hormone Replacement Therapy - Your Questions Answered." In this booklet they published the conclusions of the Committee of the Canadian Consensus on Menopause and Osteoporosis, which we have outlined below, bolding the sections that really speak to your right to choose:

- Lifestyle changes such as diet, exercise, stress reduction and quitting smoking can benefit women's emotional and physical health at midlife.
- Unless there is a medical reason for using a particular HRT delivery method, **women should decide which HRT delivery system they prefer**.

- If they wish to do so, **women should play a major role in making decisions about HRT** and other midlife health issues.

- Because HRT may slightly increase a woman's risk of developing breast cancer, **women who do decide to use HRT should have regular follow-up examinations with their doctor to reassess their need for HRT.**

- Decisions about menopausal healthcare should be based on an **individual assessment of symptoms, risk factors and the risk and benefits of possible treatments**. A woman and her healthcare professional should re-evaluate these decisions yearly and when new medical information becomes available.

Everything we have suggested and discussed in this book is consistent with the Canadian Consensus on Menopause and Osteoporosis recommendations. Women *should* be able to choose creams and patches over oral hormones. Women *should* get to play a major role in making decisions about their own healthcare. You're the one living in your body; you're the best judge of what you need! Women *should* assess their symptoms, their hormone levels, and their likelihood of developing menopause related diseases. These are the agreed upon criteria for determining whether hormone replacement is necessary. Granted there is controversy over the type of hormones to use, and the long-term risks and benefits. It *should* be apparent that bio-identical *human* hormones are a good choice, but bio-identical hormones got a slow start, perhaps because they couldn't be patented by the big drug companies. All that is changing now, and there are some commercially available bio-identical hormone options. At the very least, choose those! If you have the option, by all means explore custom compounded bio-identical hormones. Compounding pharmacists have extensive knowledge about bio-identical hormones, and hormone testing, and can act as an invaluable HRT resource for you.

There are many excellent books on the subject, and we have included a list in Resources. The more you know about hormones, the better position you're in to insist that your doctor work with you to explore hormone balance issues. There is uncertainty in all quarters. All we know for sure is that the approach we have been using carries unacceptable risks, risks that can likely be *avoided* by following nature's blueprint. We have shown you a path: now it's up to you to follow it. Good luck, and don't give up!

CHAPTER NINE

Male Hormone Balance

This chapter is our response to all those women who are worried that their men might be unbalanced. Of course, we're talking strictly about hormones here! In the words of one frustrated woman: "Now that *my* hormones are fixed, can't you please do something about my husband?" Ladies, we hear your frustration! A number of women felt we had overlooked a big piece of the hormone puzzle by not including male hormone balance in the first edition of "You've Hit Menopause: Now What?", so we decided to remedy that oversight. This chapter is here to guide you in helping the important men in your life understand how their health is impacted by hormone balance.

Most of us automatically think of testosterone when we think about male hormones. However, as you learned in the earlier chapters of this book, hormone health invariably involves more than one hormone. We want to focus your attention on how the interaction between the various hormones impacts men's health.

MALE MENOPAUSE or ANDROPAUSE?

The phrase *male menopause* often conjures up images of hairpieces and expensive sports cars, but these are not normal consequences of hormone imbalance! The terms male menopause and andropause both refer to the physical and psychological symptoms associated with a drop in androgen levels, the hormone group to which testosterone belongs. For the sake of consistency, we will use the term andropause throughout the chapter, although technically there is no *pause* in androgen production; it's more like a slow leak!

The International Society for the Study of the Aging Male defines andropause as: "A clinical and biochemical syndrome associated with advancing age and characterized by a deficiency in serum androgen levels…. It may result in significant alterations in the quality of life and adversely affect the function of multiple organ systems." In other words, the drop in androgen levels associated with aging can have a negative impact on a man's health.

The male experience of hormone decline is very different from that of women. When women reach menopause, their hormone levels drop like a rock off a cliff. For men, the hormone decline is more like a gentle roll down a hill. As a consequence, symptoms tend to appear much more gradually for men, and the women in their lives may notice the telltale signs first. Psychological symptoms may include anxiety, grumpiness, loss of interest in previously enjoyed activities, and impaired memory. Physical symptoms can include bone loss, loss of muscle strength and erectile dysfunction. The gradual nature of symptom onset has had the unfortunate consequence of causing many men to have their complaints dismissed as just being a part of aging.

So, why is testosterone so important, and what impact do other hormones have on testosterone and male health? A discussion of male hormones and the changes in hormone balance that occur at andropause provides some insight into that question.

HORMONE CHANGES IN ANDROPAUSE

The word androgen literally means 'of masculine origin'. In other words, the androgenic hormones are the hormones responsible for producing male characteristics. The most prominent androgens are testosterone and dihydro-testosterone (DHT). This section focuses primarily on the role of testosterone in andropause; therefore the other androgens will only be discussed briefly. There are several excellent books listed in the resource section at the back of this book that look at the role of androgens in the aging male in more detail.

Figure 6 shows what happens to testosterone released by the testes. In particular, it is important to note how testosterone can be 'drained off' or lost via conversion to estrogens. This can happen whether the testosterone comes from the testes or is being supplemented. The importance of this conversion will become clearer when the relationship between testosterone and estrogens is discussed later in the chapter.

Androgens

Testosterone

In men, the testes produce approximately 95% of testosterone, with the remainder coming from the adrenal glands (see Figure 3 in Chapter Two). Testosterone is primarily responsible for secondary male characteristics like: facial and body hair growth, deepening of the voice, sperm production, ability to sustain an erection, and the pubertal growth surge of the penis, prostate and scrotum. Testosterone in adult males helps provide a sense of wellbeing, control blood sugar, improve sex drive, is involved in heart health, and helps maintain skin elasticity and muscle mass. Testosterone is most active on androgen receptors found in the brain, heart and skeletal muscle.

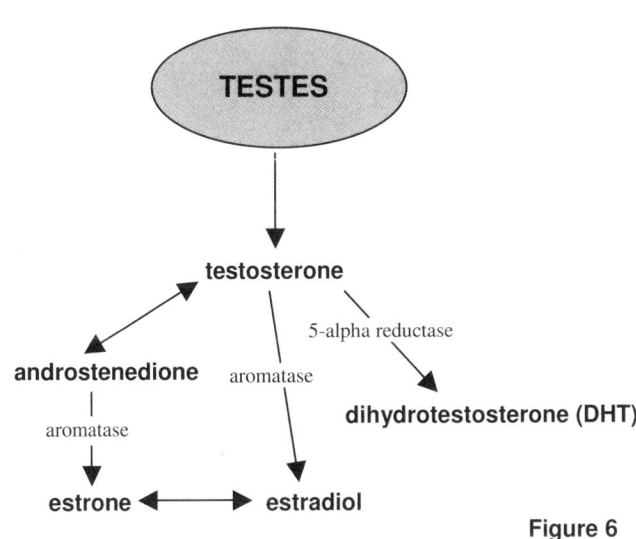

Figure 6

121

Many factors contribute to androgen decline in andropause. First, testicular production of testosterone may decrease due to an age-related decrease in the number of Leydig cells (testosterone-producing cells in the testes). Another major factor in the progression of andropause is an increase in sex hormone binding globulin (SHBG) levels (see inset below). SHBG levels increase with age and with high estradiol levels. SHBG attaches to testosterone molecules and prevents them from interacting with testosterone receptors. This means that total testosterone levels may measure normal, but the actual amount of testosterone available to cells is greatly reduced.

Sex Hormone Binding Globulin (SHBG)

Not all the testosterone in the body is available to act on androgen receptors. Some testosterone is tightly bound to a protein called Sex Hormone Binding Globulin or SHBG. Hormones bound to SHBG are too large to enter cells and are therefore unable to interact with receptors. Approximately 50% of total testosterone is tightly bound to SHBG.

Many factors influence the production of SHBG.

SHBG increases with:
- alcoholic cirrhosis
- other severe liver disease
- high levels of estrogen
- excessively high thyroid hormone levels
- age

Increased SHBG results in a decrease in the amount of free testosterone.

Total testosterone refers to the measurable amount of testosterone in the blood. However, as mentioned above, not all of this testosterone is available to tissues. About 2% of total testosterone exists in the free, unbound form in serum, while another 48% is loosely attached to a protein called albumin.

Total Testosterone

Free T	Albumin–Bound Testosterone	SHBG-Bound Testosterone

Bio-available Testosterone   **Figure 7**

Figure 7 shows the relative amounts of each form of testosterone. The combination of free testosterone and albumin-bound testosterone is called *bio-available* testosterone (see inset below).

Free versus Bio-Available Testosterone

Free testosterone is testosterone that is not bound to any proteins and is free to act on hormone receptors.

Some testosterone binds loosely to the protein albumin. Albumin is present in large quantities in the blood, and albumin-bound testosterone detaches easily and becomes free testosterone. In other words, albumin serves as a kind of reservoir for testosterone. This is called *bio-available* testosterone, because it is testosterone that is *available* to testosterone receptors in tissue.

The decline in both free and bio-available testosterone levels with age is well documented. *Bio-available* testosterone drops by approximately 1% per year after age 40. Around age 40, only one or two men out of a hundred have subnormal testosterone levels, but by age 60, one out of every five men has subnormal testosterone. Comparing the *free* testosterone levels of young adults and seniors reveals that 70-year old men have less than half the free testosterone levels of 25-year olds.

In addition, some men may suffer from a *relative* lack of testosterone. These are men who had higher than average testosterone levels in their youth and have normal (compared to their peers) levels of free or bio-available testosterone later in life, but now this normal testosterone level *seems* too low. Their bodies are used to higher levels of testosterone, and perceive the drop in testosterone (even though it is still in the normal range) as a deficiency. They are said to be suffering from a *relative* lack of testosterone because they have too little testosterone relative to the levels of their youth.

Symptoms of low bio-available testosterone or androgen deficiency include fatigue, decreased sex drive, diminished quality of erections, as well as worsening of athletic performance, strength and endurance. Other symptoms may include loss of self-esteem, depression, irritability, loss of motivation and overall decreased enjoyment of life.

Symptoms of androgen excess include acne, irritability and oily skin. Progesterone slows down the enzyme that converts testosterone into its more potent form, dihydrotestosterone or DHT. Some men supplement with progesterone to reduce formation of DHT and reduce symptoms of androgen excess.

Dihydrotestosterone (DHT)

The enzyme 5-alpha-reductase converts testosterone into dihydrotestosterone (see Figure 6, page 122). DHT is approximately ten times more active than testosterone. This means DHT binds ten times more strongly to androgen receptors than testosterone. DHT is most active in the skin, prostate and seminal glands. DHT has relatively little effect on brain tissues. DHT is often blamed for conditions of androgen excess like male-pattern baldness, acne, and facial and body hair growth.

Androgens

Deficiency	Excess
Low sex drive	Irritability
Feel "burned out"	Increased aggressiveness
Decreased endurance	Oily skin
Fatigue	Increased acne
Muscle aches/stiffness	Increased stroke risk
Depression	High cholesterol
Bone loss	Increased proportion of red
Decreased muscle mass	blood cells in blood
Decreased erections	(hematocrit)
Loss of morning erection	
Penis shrinkage	
Loss of sense of humour	
Grumpiness	
Increased sweating	
Lack of enthusiasm	

Table 6

DHEA and Androstenedione

Dehydroepiandrosterone (DHEA) is the most abundant steroid hormone in the body and is the primary building block for androgens. DHEA levels decline with age and this decline can be linked to a general decrease in quality of life. Symptoms like decreased energy and motivation, inability to cope and emotional numbing and sadness may be associated with low DHEA and/or DHEA-sulphate (the main type of DHEA circulating in blood) levels. Lower DHEA levels also accompany chronic illnesses such as lupus, rheumatoid arthritis, multiple sclerosis, AIDS and hepatitis.

DHEA and cortisol have opposite effects on immune function and regulation of blood sugar. For example, DHEA can improve sensitivity to insulin, which helps to lower blood glucose levels. Conversely, cortisol *increases* blood glucose levels. An excess of cortisol relative to DHEA has also been linked to poorer performance on standard tests designed to evaluate memory and judgment (cognitive function tests). When cortisol levels are too high, DHEA must be released to balance the effects of the cortisol. Consequently, chronically elevated cortisol levels can result in a deficiency of DHEA. Hormone testing should include both cortisol and DHEA or DHEAS in order to determine whether the two are in balance.

Androstenedione is made from DHEA in the adrenal glands and is a precursor to both estrogens and testosterone. Although androgens are usually the main focus of any discussion of andropause, it is very important to examine the interaction between estrogens and androgens. An understanding of the relationship between these two hormone groups is essential to any examination of andropause issues.

Estrogens

Maintaining a balance between androgens and estrogen is crucial to good health. Estrogen receptors in men are found in the testes, bone, brain, blood vessels, bladder, breast, and thyroid gland. Although there are three main estrogens: estradiol, estrone and estriol, this chapter focuses primarily on estradiol, the strongest of the three. The testes produce approximately 20% of a man's estradiol while most of the remaining estradiol is made in body fat from androgens via the enzyme aromatase. Figure 6 shows how the aromatase enzyme converts the androgens androstenedione and testosterone into estrogens. Aromatase is found in fat cells, so overweight men or men with extra fat around the waist have more of this enzyme, and are therefore likely to make more estrogen.

Other factors promoting estrogen excess include zinc deficiency, excessive consumption of commercially raised beef and poultry (see xenoestrogens page 23), constipation (reduces elimination of estrogens) and excessive alcohol intake. Supplements like DHEA, growth hormone releasing agents and boron can also elevate estrogens. Table 7 shows the symptoms associated with high estrogen levels in men.

Estrogens can compete directly with testosterone at the receptor site, thereby weakening the effects of testosterone, even if the testosterone level is normal. Higher estrogen levels may also increase SHBG, which ties up testosterone so it can't be delivered to tissue.

Estrogens	
Deficiency	**Excess**
Hot flashes	Breast enlargement
Night sweats	Weight gain (hips)
Bone loss	Low sex drive
Memory problems	Enlarged prostate
	Increased urge to urinate
	Decreased urine flow
	Cold body temperature

Table 7

Nutritional deficiency may also contribute to higher estrogen levels. As we age, we become less able to liberate and absorb trace minerals from our food. Zinc is a critically important trace mineral for men, as it helps block the conversion of androgens to estrogens; therefore a zinc deficiency could lead to symptoms of low testosterone.

Cortisol

The role of cortisol in normal physiology was discussed in Chapter Two. Although not directly involved in the evolution of andropause, cortisol is crucial for two reasons: it can interfere with the actions of other hormones (i.e. androgens and thyroid hormone) and it can increase aromatase-induced conversion of testosterone into estradiol. Poorly managed stress raises cortisol, which 'turns on' the aromatase enzyme.

Cortisol

Deficiency	Excess
Fatigue	Irritability
Allergies	'Tired but wired' feeling
Aching muscles	Weight gain - waist
Feeling cold	Loss of muscle mass
Neck stiffness	Bone loss
Increased infections	High blood pressure
Morning sluggishness	Insulin resistance
'Burned out' feeling	Low sex drive
Low sex drive	Impaired memory
Feel unable to cope	Loss of scalp hair
	'Burned out' feeling
	Depression

Table 8

Cortisol also promotes fat deposition around the waist, which increases the size of the "factory" where aromatase enzyme makes estrogen. Many troublesome symptoms for men actually have their roots in a deficiency or excess of cortisol. The symptoms associated with cortisol excess or deficiency are the same for men and women, and although listed earlier in the book, are repeated in Table 8.

HORMONE INTERACTIONS

Androgens, Estrogens and Cortisol

The balance between testosterone, estradiol and cortisol in men is vital. Hormone imbalances can lead to symptoms of low testosterone, even if testosterone levels are normal. This type of problem is called a functional deficiency. The testosterone level may be normal, but the system *functions* as if testosterone were low. Functional testosterone deficiency can arise when either cortisol or estrogen levels are higher than normal. Both estradiol and cortisol can compete with testosterone at the receptor level.

Estradiol and testosterone try to occupy the same receptor, like two people trying to fit through a doorway at the same time. Thus, when estradiol levels are high, they occupy more receptor sites and prevent testosterone from reaching the receptor. The testosterone is available, but unable to act on the receptor. Over time, the brain can interpret high estradiol levels as a sign that testosterone is too high, and may issue instructions to decrease production, thereby creating an *actual* deficiency of testosterone.

Cortisol and testosterone deliver opposite messages through the same receptor. As discussed in Chapter Two, testosterone builds up muscle while cortisol breaks it down. Thus, high levels of cortisol can directly oppose the message testosterone is trying to deliver, even if there is adequate testosterone available. Research on military recruits showed that in the face of acute stress, elevated cortisol was accompanied by a significant drop in testosterone. Therefore, what starts out as a *functional* deficiency could evolve into an *actual* deficiency, with measurably low testosterone levels. The important message here is that men may have normal levels of testosterone, but have too much estradiol or cortisol *relative* to testosterone.

Ratio of Testosterone to Estradiol

A good way to assess the potential for functional deficiency is to examine the ratio of testosterone to estradiol. Consider Moe, a 50-year old male complaining of low sex drive and fatigue. He recently had salivary hormone testing done, with the following results:

Testosterone (T) level   50 pg/ml (normal)
Estradiol   (E2) level   3.5 pg/ml (normal)

Despite the fact that testosterone and estradiol fall within the normal observed range, Moe is suffering some classic symptoms of testosterone deficiency. A look at the ratio of testosterone to estradiol reveals the reason. A laboratory survey of men under thirty-five years of age showed that more than nine out of ten men have a ratio of testosterone to estradiol between 20 and 40. In Moe's case, his ratio of T to E2 was 14, well below the normal range. Moe's low T:E2 ratio indicates that he has too much estrogen (estradiol) relative to testosterone or not enough testosterone relative to estradiol, even though both hormones are in the normal range.

Further investigation reveals that Moe is under a lot of stress at work, is 35 pounds overweight, loves red meat, drinks three or four beers each night and sports a substantial 'spare tire'! In all likelihood, it is these lifestyle factors that have created Moe's imbalance between testosterone and estradiol.

Excess alcohol intake and frequent consumption of commercially raised beef can both increase estrogen levels. Moe is under a lot of stress and stress elevates cortisol, which can create abdominal fat deposits and 'turn on' the aromatase enzyme that converts testosterone to estradiol.

Further saliva testing reveals that Moe's morning cortisol is indeed higher than normal.

In the final analysis, Moe needs to lose weight, eat less red meat, eat hormone-free meat and poultry, and reduce his alcohol consumption in order to bring down his estrogen levels. He also needs to learn how to manage stress better so he can bring his cortisol levels down. Testosterone supplementation is unlikely to benefit Moe, because much of his testosterone is being converted to estradiol. In other words, testosterone supplementation could actually *worsen* Moe's symptoms of testosterone deficiency!

Thyroid Hormone Interactions

The importance of thyroid hormone is often overlooked in discussions of male hormone balance. Free testosterone levels can be influenced by thyroid hormone. For example, an overactive thyroid (hyperthyroidism) can decrease SHBG levels, which results in an increase in free testosterone (see inset page 123). Conversely, an underactive thyroid (hypothyroidism) can increase SHBG and result in decreased free testosterone levels.

Excess estrogen can also adversely affect thyroid function and result in symptoms of hypothyroidism. In such cases, thyroid hormone levels may be normal, but the presence of excess estrogens interferes with the action of the thyroid hormone.

And last, though definitely not least, cortisol is a critical component in thyroid hormone function. Cortisol and thyroid hormones have a mutually dependent relationship: a certain amount of thyroid hormone is needed for cortisol to work properly, and a certain amount of cortisol is necessary for thyroid hormones to work properly. As a result, an excess of thyroid hormone can impair the activity of cortisol and vice versa.

The complex interplay between hormones and the failure to maintain the right balance of hormones may lead to some of the symptoms and diseases associated with andropause. The next section provides some insights into the relationship between symptoms, disease states and hormone imbalance.

SYMPTOMS

There are a number of characteristic symptoms associated with male hormone imbalance. The following is a guide to some of the more common symptoms, along with a brief description of the hormone imbalances that may be contributing to those symptoms.

Breast enlargement: Men with extra weight around the middle have more aromatase and therefore convert more testosterone into estradiol. Excess estrogens can lead to breast enlargement.

Depression or grumpiness: The brain is rich in androgen receptors, and therefore low androgen levels will have an effect on brain function. Depression, grumpiness and/or loss of interest in new things are common symptoms of low testosterone.

Erectile dysfunction: Androgen receptors are abundant in the brain and testosterone, the main androgen, plays an important part in the arousal response. A lack of testosterone may reduce the arousal response, and result in difficulties achieving an erection. Although testosterone is only one factor in producing and maintaining an erection, it is a key player in the process. Low testosterone levels may be associated with a longer 'wait' time to achieve erection. Reduction in testosterone can also affect the muscle surrounding the urethra and the bladder. With insufficient testosterone, the muscle contracts less efficiently, which can lead to decreased erection quality. Low testosterone may also result in penis shrinkage.

Loss of muscle mass: Testosterone is the hormone responsible for building and maintaining muscle mass, so low testosterone can lead to lost muscle mass. High cortisol levels also contribute to loss of muscle mass.

Memory loss: The presence of testosterone receptors in the brain means that decreases in testosterone will affect the brain. This often manifests itself as memory loss.

Weight gain: There are a number of hormone issues associated with weight gain. Men with high cortisol levels will tend to maintain more weight around the middle (central obesity). The irony is, some men think it's macho to have a beer belly, but in fact, it makes them more feminine! The fatter they are, the more aromatase they have, which converts testosterone to estradiol. The increase in estradiol and decrease in testosterone contributes to decreased muscle mass and a tendency to gain more weight around the middle, a self-perpetuating cycle of hormone imbalance. Central obesity also increases a man's risk of developing heart disease and diabetes.

HORMONE IMBALANCE AND DISEASE

Heart Disease and Diabetes: Figure 8 illustrates how imbalances between testosterone, estradiol and cortisol can contribute to the development of heart disease and diabetes.

Low levels of free testosterone are associated with both heart disease and diabetes. High levels of estradiol contribute to heart disease, while diabetes contributes to

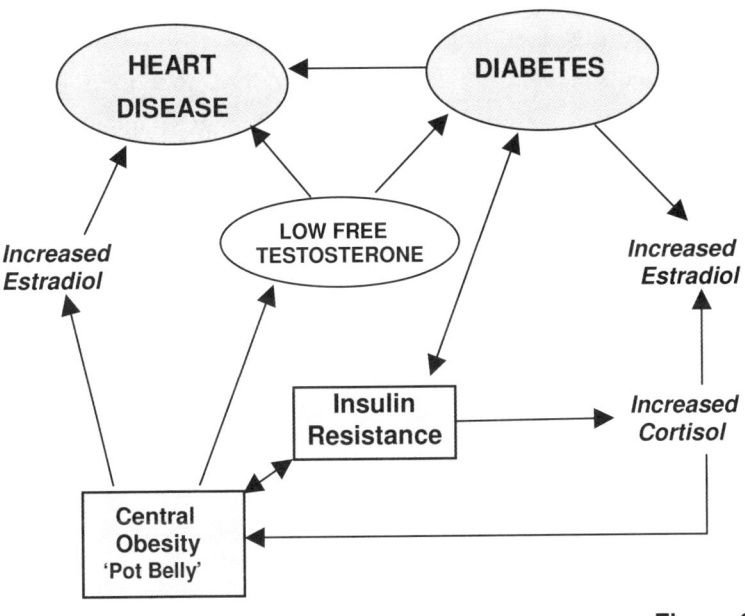

Figure 8

higher levels of estradiol. This is one reason why men with diabetes are at higher risk of developing heart disease. High cortisol levels also increase estradiol levels and can contribute to central obesity, which in turn can increase the risk of heart disease.

Figure 8 highlights the importance of maintaining the right balance between hormones to prevent heart disease and diabetes. However, there are a number of other diseases that are impacted by hormone imbalance:

Benign Prostatic Hyperplasia (BPH): This condition is extremely common in the aging male. Most men over the age of sixty have some signs of prostate enlargement, although not all have symptoms. Some researchers believe BPH might be a result of low testosterone or high estradiol. This theory is partially based on the fact that men with declining testosterone levels have the highest incidence of BPH, while men in their peak testosterone producing years have an extremely low incidence of BPH. Also, since the prostate is derived from the same tissue as the uterus in the embryo stage, researchers believe that excessive estrogen exposure may result in overgrowth of the prostate.

Breast Cancer: Although breast cancer in men is rare, men with too much estrogen relative to testosterone are at greater risk of developing breast cancer. Both obesity and liver disease can contribute to excess estrogens in men.

Osteoporosis: Low testosterone or low estradiol can both contribute to osteoporosis. Testosterone is the hormone primarily responsible for building bone mass in men. High cortisol levels can also accelerate the breakdown of bone.

Prostate cancer: Men with normal testosterone levels at the time of prostate cancer diagnosis have a better survival rate than men with low testosterone levels. However, once prostate cancer has been diagnosed, testosterone should not be supplemented as it may accelerate tumour growth. Low levels of DHT relative to testosterone have also been associated with prostate cancer.

PROSTATE SPECIFIC ANTIGEN (PSA)

The PSA, or prostate-specific antigen level in the blood, is commonly used as a marker for increased risk of prostate cancer. When PSA levels are above a certain threshold prostate cancer is suspected and a biopsy of the prostate may be warranted.

Hormone imbalance can be a contributing factor in many of the major causes of death for men, so restoring the right balance is essential to achieving and maintaining good health. However, it is impossible to restore hormone balance without first knowing what is out of balance. Hormone testing is the only sure way to find out whether a hormone imbalance is present.

HORMONE TESTING FOR MEN

A key factor in testing is the need to measure the amount of bio-available testosterone, not just the total testosterone. (see inset page 124)   As described earlier in this chapter, the total testosterone level can be quite misleading, as it can remain relatively constant throughout life, even though the amount of testosterone available to cells steadily declines.

Both blood and saliva tests are commonly used to test for testosterone. A description of the pros and cons of each method follows.

Blood

Some laboratories offer a test called the Free Androgen Index (FAI). The FAI is not an actual hormone level, but is a calculated value that approximates the amount of bio-available testosterone in blood. To generate the FAI, the laboratory measures total testosterone and SHBG (see inset page 123). The following formula is then used to calculate the amount of testosterone available to tissues:

$$\text{Free Androgen Index} = \frac{\text{Total Testosterone}}{\text{SHBG}} \times 100$$

Bioavailable testosterone in blood can also be measured via a technique known as equilibrium dialysis, which is often regarded as the 'gold standard' (most widely accepted) way of measuring bio-available testosterone.

Free testosterone (not bound to either albumin or SHBG) can be measured separately in blood by several methods, but is only available through certain laboratories.

Ultimately, the Free Androgen Index, equilibrium dialysis and free testosterone all involve a trip to a laboratory to have blood drawn, which can be inconvenient. On the other hand, blood tests *may* be paid for by government-funded health insurance plans, at least for the time being. In this climate of health care cost-cutting, it is quite likely that hormone testing will come under scrutiny eventually, since some people consider testing hormones medically unnecessary!

Saliva

Because hormones must pass through tissue (the saliva gland) to get into saliva, saliva testing is an excellent measure of the amount of testosterone that actually gets to tissue. Saliva testing compares very favourably to the 'gold standard' test for bio-available testosterone in blood.

Another factor to consider is that testosterone levels are highest in the morning, and decline throughout the day. A blood sample taken later in the day may read low simply because the normal range was based on early morning blood samples. Since saliva testing is done at home, a sample can easily be taken within the first hour of waking, ensuring a result that can be compared to the normal morning range. This is not always convenient or possible with blood tests.

In addition, saliva is well on its way to becoming the gold standard test for cortisol. The prospect of having blood drawn may cause cortisol levels to rise, and so cortisol levels in blood may appear artificially high. Estrogens are also commonly and reliably tested in saliva.

HORMONE REPLACEMENT FOR MEN

If hormone testing reveals a hormone imbalance, some kind of intervention will be required. Clearly, not all men with symptoms of low testosterone need to supplement with testosterone. If issues like high estradiol and cortisol are identified, then lifestyle changes should be initiated. An exercise regimen, healthy eating, and stress management are all important lifestyle goals. Undiagnosed sleep problems like sleep apnea can also feed into hormone imbalance. Men with sleep apnea have been shown to have lower testosterone levels; therefore a careful sleep history is essential to any inquiry into andropause complaints.

Ultimately though, there are many men who are likely to benefit from supplementing with testosterone. Hopefully, their physicians will agree that a trial of testosterone replacement is warranted when testing confirms the need.

Currently, men have a wide range of options for prescription bio-identical testosterone replacement; either ready made or made-to-order by compounding pharmacists, and these products are listed in Table 9.

	Ready made products	**Custom compounds**
Oral	**Andriol®** (testosterone undeconate)	Micronized **testosterone** capsules, troches, sublingual drops
Injectable	**Delatestryl®** (testosterone cypionate)	n/a
Skin patch	**Androderm®**	n/a
Topical skin product	**Androgel®**	**testosterone** cream or gel

Table 9

As discussed in Chapter Four, delivery of hormones through skin is most efficient. The administered dose of testosterone remains unchanged (stays as testosterone) much longer when it is given through the skin, avoiding immediate breakdown or conversion into other hormones like estradiol. Testosterone patches are an excellent way to deliver testosterone. Their main drawback is that they only come in two strengths, meaning it is difficult to change the dose to meet an individual's specific needs. Compounded topical testosterone is preferred by many patients and practitioners, since it allows precise control of dosing, and the amount of product applied to the skin can be as little as 0.1 ml. Androgel®, a commercially available gel, comes in 5 gram packets, and many men find it inconvenient to apply this much product (roughly one teaspoonful).

Testosterone injections result in wide swings in the amount of testosterone available to the body: too much or just enough immediately after the injection, and too little before the next injection is due. Also, testosterone is normally highest in the morning, and declines throughout the day. This physiologic pattern can be mimicked with oral or skin delivered testosterone, but is lost when testosterone is only injected once every two weeks or so.

A young man naturally produces about 5 mg of testosterone per day. Therefore, testosterone delivered through the skin should be in the range of 2 to 5 mg per day. As described in Chapter Four, taking hormones orally is very inefficient, and therefore higher doses tend to be used.

It is tempting for practitioners to chase testosterone-related symptoms with ever-increasing doses of testosterone. However, if physiologic doses of testosterone do not relieve symptoms, the practitioner, pharmacist and patient need to step back and reassess the situation: a switch to a different delivery system may be indicated along with consideration of other factors such as estrogen and cortisol levels.

Unlike women, whose hormone production varies throughout the month, men produce roughly the same amount of testosterone each day. Therefore, in theory, testosterone should be given every morning. However, in practice, to avoid loss of effectiveness, testosterone 'holidays' are often incorporated into the dosing schedule. For example; six days on, one day off; three weeks on, three days off, and so forth.

Overdose can also lead to loss of effectiveness, since receptors will down-regulate or 'turn off' because the hormone 'signal' is too loud. If a previously effective dose stops working, this may indicate a need for a dose reduction, a change in the dosing schedule, or perhaps a two to four week break from therapy to allow the body to regain its sensitivity to testosterone.

CASE STUDIES

The following case studies illustrate some of the more common issues associated with hormone replacement in men.

RALPH

History

Ralph is 64 years old and complains of a gradual decline in energy, increased apathy, decreased sex drive, mild depression and irritability. His wife has noticed a decrease in the (flaccid) size of his penis and a decrease in the size of his testicles. His PSA (see inset page 138) is normal and on physical examination, his prostate feels normal.

Symptom Analysis

Ralph's symptoms suggest testosterone deficiency.

Saliva Hormone Test Results

Estradiol: 2 pg/ml   (normal)
Testosterone: 35 pg/ml (low normal)
T/E2:   *17.5*   (low) *20 to 40 desirable*
DHEAS: 5 ng/ml   (normal)
Cortisol: 5.3 ng/ml (normal)

Saliva Test Interpretation

Testosterone is low normal. The ratio of testosterone to estradiol, T/E2, is low. Ralph has a classic pattern of isolated low testosterone. Adrenal hormone output is normal.

Recommendations for Ralph

Since there is no clinical or laboratory indication of prostate cancer, and provided there are no other medical contra-indications such as liver disease or clotting disorder, Ralph might be a good candidate for a trial of testosterone replacement with a starting dose of 1 to 2 mg transdermally, once each morning. His PSA (see inset page 138), hematocrit, lipid parameters and liver function will be monitored periodically by his family physician. (There is no evidence that physiologic, transdermal doses of testosterone have a negative effect on liver function. However, excessive prolonged use of synthetic, so-called 'anabolic steroids' such as those used by athletes and bodybuilders may be harmful to the liver.)

MOE
History

We discussed Moe in detail earlier in the chapter. His is a typical case of functional testosterone deficiency. His testosterone level is fine, but his symptoms are mainly the result of interference by high estrogen and high cortisol. The best solution to Moe's problem involves lifestyle changes. Some physicians are also using aromatase inhibitors such as Femara® (starting with very small doses like 0.5 mg twice weekly) in patients like Moe to block the conversion of testosterone to estradiol.

DAVID
History

David is a 52-year-old man who started testosterone replacement (compounded testosterone cream) six years ago, after blood and saliva testing confirmed low bioavailable testosterone. He did well until recently, when his wife started supplementing with topical progesterone, 100 mg per day. She usually rubs the progesterone cream on her breasts each evening. Now he complains of hot flashes, increased sweating, and a loss of sex drive.

Symptom Analysis

David's symptoms suggest testosterone deficiency.

Saliva Hormone Test Results

Estradiol: 3 pg/ml (normal)

Testosterone: 800 pg/ml (normal for topical supplement)

Progesterone: 3350 pg/ml (high)

Saliva Test Interpretation

This is a very interesting case. David is being exposed to progesterone through skin-to-skin contact with his wife! Since progesterone blocks the conversion of testosterone to its more potent derivative, dihydrotestosterone, it has the potential to reduce the efficacy of testosterone replacement therapy.

Recommendations for David

David and his wife Jocelyn need to co-ordinate their intimate activities so that he avoids exposure to her progesterone.   Jocelyn might consider applying the progesterone earlier in the evening, then taking a shower before bed. She might also want to revisit her dosing, as 100 mg is an excessive dose for topical progesterone.

LARRY

History

Larry is 48 years old, and started testosterone replacement with Androgel®, one packet per day, two months ago. It worked well initially, but lately he feels like it has quit working. He has also noticed some breast enlargement.

Symptom Analysis

Larry's symptoms suggest estrogen excess.

Saliva Hormone Test Results

Estradiol: 8 pg/ml (high)

Testosterone: >1200 pg/ml (high)

Saliva Test Interpretation

Both estradiol and testosterone are above their expected ranges. One packet of Androgel® contains 50mg of testosterone, 10 times more than the average amount produced by an 18 year old male! The excess testosterone is 'spilling over' to estradiol. Furthermore, Larry's receptors are no longer 'listening' to the testosterone message, because it is too loud, and has been delivered at the same intensity for too long.

Recommendations for Larry

Larry needs to stop testosterone therapy for one to two months, to give his body time to "reset" itself. Testosterone therapy can then be restarted with a more physiologic dose, something closer to the normal daily production of 5mg. Consideration might also be given to introduction of scheduled breaks in the therapy, such as one day off per week, or several consecutive days off per month.

CONCLUSION

It has been estimated that over one million Canadian men suffer from a testosterone deficiency and that only 5% currently receive treatment! Imbalances between the various sex hormones can cause significant health problems in men, just as they can for women.

There is good evidence that adequate testosterone is protective against diseases of the heart and blood vessels, and several researchers have suggested that it may be protective against prostate cancer as well. Low testosterone has been associated with depression, while excessive amounts of testosterone have been linked to aggression. Low testosterone and high estradiol have been associated with increased risk of diabetes. Research also shows that proper hormone balance is essential to a healthy immune system. Clearly hormones have a significant role to play in maintaining men's health!

Unfortunately, some critics have used the negative press around female hormone replacement therapy (HRT) to condemn testosterone replacement therapy for men. They claim that the negative results found with use of synthetic hormones in women prove that giving men testosterone is a bad idea. In fact, these studies only proved that *non-human* hormones do not provide health benefits. Male hormone replacement therapy already has a huge advantage over female HRT in that men almost always receive bio-identical testosterone. In 2003, leading Canadian urologist Dr. Alvaro Morales stated: "Recent concerns about HRT in postmenopausal women have been inappropriately extrapolated to men by the lay press. Such extrapolation is not only inappropriate but it lacks any scientific evidence or validity." In other words, it's unreasonable and unscientific to say that because female hormone replacement studies using non-identical hormones showed negative results that men should be denied hormone replacement!

Although it is impossible for one chapter to cover the whole topic of male hormone replacement in detail, we hope we have given women, and the important men in their lives, a place to start. As is true for women, collaboration between the male patient, his physician, and a compounding pharmacist will lead to the best possible outcome. Women need to have the *all* the hormone facts, not just for themselves, but also for the important men in their lives. Make hormone balance a family affair!

APPENDIX A

Bio-Identical Hormone Products

Bio-identical hormone replacement and compounding pharmacy go hand-in-hand. Compounding refers to the art of custom preparation of medicines. The origins of the profession of pharmacy are rooted in the preparation of custom tonics, ointments and herbal remedies. The introduction of manufactured pharmaceuticals drastically reduced the need for compounded prescriptions. At first, bio-identical hormones were not available commercially as they were not well absorbed. Advances in manufacturing have resolved these early problems and now bio-identical hormones are readily available in commercially manufactured products. Transdermal estradiol patches and gels are common examples of commercially available bio-identical hormones.

Limited dose and delivery system options with commercially manufactured products may lead to poor therapeutic results for some people. Customization of the dose and delivery system for specific needs is easier to achieve with pharmaceutical compounding. In consultation with your physician, specialized compounding pharmacies (see Resources) can customize a hormone prescription to your specific needs. Most of these compounding pharmacists belong to organizations dedicated to continuing education and excellence in all areas of compounding but particularly bio-identical hormone replacement.

Estrogens

TriEst (or triple estrogen) is a compounded product consisting of differing ratios of estradiol, estrone and estriol. TriEst was originally formulated based on research suggesting that estriol present in 10-fold excess over estradiol might provide estrogenic effects without increasing the risk of cancer. A paper published several years ago measured the levels of these three estrogens in blood and claimed to show that estriol was the most abundant estrogen in blood. Unfortunately, this research was flawed and therefore does not support a formulation in which estriol is the most abundant estrogen. The amount of each type of estrogen in the formulation should be determined primarily by the patient's symptoms and risk of disease (e.g. breast cancer and osteoporosis). The dose or strength of the TriEst capsule is expressed as total milligrams of estrogen (the combination of estriol, estrone and estradiol), and the ratio of the hormones is also indicated. It is can be compounded into either capsule or cream form. The commonly used strengths of TriEst are 1.25mg. 2.5mg and 5.0mg. There are many ratios possible, but the following are some of the formulations commonly seen by compounding pharmacists.

- 80:10:10   1.25mg capsule = 1mg estriol + 0.125mg estrone + 0.125 mg estradiol

- 70:20:10   1.25 mg capsule = 0.875 mg estriol + 0.25mg estrone + 0.125mg E2
- 90:5:5   1.25 mg = 1.125 mg estriol + 0.0625 mg estrone + 0.0625mg estradiol

BiEst eliminates estrone from the estrogen mix, leaving only estriol and estradiol. Since the body is quite capable of making estrone from estradiol, there is usually no need to give it more. Supplementing with too much estrone may result in an excess of estrone sulphate and other potentially harmful metabolites like 4-hydroxyestrone, strongly implicated in breast cancer. As for TriEst, the strength of BiEst is expressed as total milligrams of estrogens, usually 1.25mg, 2.5mg and 5.0 mg doses, and the ratio of the two hormones is indicated. The most common ratios of BiEst are:

- 80:20   80% estriol and 20% estradiol
          1.25mg = 1.0mg estriol + 0.25mg estradiol

Estriol is also given on its own. Vaginal estriol is very effective for urinary incontinence, in addition to helping relieve vaginal dryness. Sustained release estriol capsules are also prescribed to help relieve menopause symptoms in women with high breast cancer risk, or with active breast cancer. The daily dose for oral estriol varies from 0.5 mg every other day up to 5 mg daily in some cases. Saliva testing indicates that many women accumulate estriol with time. This is because it is at the end of the metabolic road. In Europe, estriol doses tend to be lower: 0.5 mg/day or every other day.

Estradiol can be compounded into any of the various delivery systems, including sustained release capsules, transdermal, topical, and vaginal creams, as well as sublingual and buccal forms. Commercially available estradiol patches are also an excellent way to deliver a steady amount of hormone and produce relatively consistent hormone levels. As described earlier in the book, delivery of hormones through the skin more closely approximates the way the body naturally distributes hormones.

Progesterone

Progesterone is commonly made into transdermal or topical creams, sustained release capsules and vaginal suppositories. Transdermal and topical progesterone formulations can be made in a variety of strengths, from less than 1% (1 gram per 100ml) all the way up to 40% or more. The usual prescribed dose of progesterone for women ranges between 20 and 40mg daily. A 2% progesterone cream delivers 20mg progesterone per ml, so this is a commonly used strength. (Progesterone creams up to 1.5% strength are available in the United States without a prescription, but the quality can vary widely. Some over-the-counter creams do not even contain progesterone.) To get an exact dose of a compounded cream, most pharmacies will supply patients with a measuring spoon or syringe. Progesterone cream can be applied to any skin areas, although the abdomen should probably be avoided. Hormone applied to the abdominal skin is delivered to the liver and broken down before it is delivered to tissue. Progesterone applied to breast tissue may help relieve the discomfort associated with fibrocystic breasts and dense breast tissue.

Progesterone is available commercially as Prometrium® 100mg capsules. Compounded sustained release capsules are usually formulated in a 100mg or 200mg strength, and the progesterone is released slowly over approximately 12 hours. Taken orally, progesterone is broken down by the liver into progesterone metabolites; therefore oral doses need to be at least 100 mg whereas skin doses are 1/5th to 1/10th as large. Progesterone metabolites cause drowsiness for some women, and also exert a tranquilizing effect. Therefore oral delivery might be more appropriate if these effects are desired.

Androgens and Androgen Precursors

Testosterone can be compounded into creams or gels, generally prepared in the range of 0.2 to 2%. Testosterone is available commercially as a transdermal patch and in gel form. The Androderm® patch is only available in 2.5mg and 5mg strengths, whereas women need only 0.5 to 1.0 mg. AndroGel® comes in a 1% strength, but is much more expensive than compounded testosterone. Andriol® capsules contain a modified form of testosterone: testosterone undecanoate. As discussed in Chapter Four, oral delivery of hormone is not ideal because the hormone is modified by the liver prior to getting to tissue.

DHEA: As of this printing, DHEA was not yet licensed as a natural product in Canada. However, a recent amendment to regulations allows natural products like DHEA to be supplied through the Special Access Program (SAP). Requests under the SAP must be made by a practitioner for a specific drug, in a specific dosage form, for a specific patient, to treat a serious illness.

Glucocorticoids

Cortisol: Severe cortisol deficiency is uncommon. It may be genetic, may arise from other diseases or may be a consequence of surgery. Chronic stress can also lead to a cortisol deficiency. Supplementation with cortisol can be helpful in allowing the adrenal glands to rest during early recovery from adrenal fatigue (see Chapter Two). Cortisol is available commercially in tablet form, and is also commonly used topically to treat minor skin rashes. It is possible to absorb enough cortisol from creams to affect the body's own production of cortisol. Consequently, overuse of cortisone-based skin creams should be avoided.

HORMONE DELIVERY SYSTEMS

There are many dosage forms available to choose from. Dosage forms are also known as *delivery systems*, because they are responsible for the way the hormone is *delivered* to tissue. We will discuss the most common delivery systems for bio-identical hormone replacement, and the potential advantages and disadvantages of each.

Oral

One of the reasons synthetic hormones were developed (aside from profit!) was that bio-identical hormones were thought to be poorly absorbed. That's no longer true and effective oral forms of bio-identical hormones are readily available.   There are some commercially available bio-identical oral hormones including Estrace® (estradiol), and Prometrium® (oral micronized progesterone). Prometrium® is formulated in peanut oil, which is a potentially serious allergen for many people. Ogen® (estropipate, a form of estrone sulphate) is also available, but excessive amounts of estrone sulphate should be avoided. Commercially available oral bio-identical hormones tend to be rapidly eliminated from the body. This has prompted compounding pharmacists to develop long acting forms of oral bio-identical hormones.   This is often accomplished by formulating the hormone with a gelatin-like substance called hydroxypropylmethylcellulose. The addition of this compound allows a gradual release of hormone throughout the day.   In theory, this sustained release action results in more consistent hormone levels throughout the day, and hormone testing seems to confirm that this actually occurs.

Advantages: Oral estradiol has been shown to increase HDL (*good* cholesterol). Many people find capsules more convenient than drops, lozenges or creams. Physicians are often more comfortable prescribing commercially available products.

Disadvantages: Studies show oral estrogens affect the natural production patterns of liver proteins. These proteins are involved in blood clotting, regulation of insulin, and delivery of cortisol and thyroid hormone to tissue. Therefore, giving estrogens orally could theoretically result in an increased tendency to clotting, poor insulin regulation and decreased thyroid function.

All orally administered hormones are subject to destruction by stomach acid and metabolism by the liver. Up to 80% of oral progesterone is converted to metabolites by the gut and also the liver; the so-called *first pass* effect. Sometimes these hormone metabolites can be useful. For example, the progesterone metabolites pregnanolone, allopregnanolone and hydroxypregnanone may cause drowsiness. Thus, given at bedtime, oral micronized progesterone (Prometrium®) can help induce sleep in women who suffer from hormone related insomnia. The longer acting compounded form of progesterone is less likely to cause drowsiness.

The magnitude of this *first pass* effect by the liver is largely responsible for the appeal of non-oral forms of hormone replacement. Delivery through the skin more closely approximates the body's own natural delivery of hormones, as it circulates hormones to tissue prior to metabolism by the liver. Even so, it is sometimes appropriate to give hormones orally.

Delivery Through Skin

The membranes around skin cells contain lipids, or fats, that help to control the entry of substances into the cell. Hormones are lipophilic or fat-loving substances and as such, are good candidates for absorption across the skin. In order for hormones to work their magic on hormone receptors in tissues, the hormone cream must pass through the layers of skin. The first layer, the stratum corneum, forms a protective barrier and is generally the strongest obstacle to penetration. Hormones then pass through the rest of the epidermis and into the dermis. Once in the dermis, hormone may be delivered to the adipose (fat) cells, or to the small blood vessels (capillaries). Where the hormone winds up may depend on the delivery system used.

There are two ways of delivering hormones through skin: transdermal and topical. Bases are the creams or gels that the hormones are mixed into. Transdermal delivery involves the use of chemical absorption enhancers in the base to enable hormones to penetrate deep into the dermis and enter the capillaries. In contrast, topical creams avoid using penetration enhancers, and hormones likely only get as far as the adipose cells. It has been argued that the enhancers in transdermal bases may result in faster elimination of hormones than the topical creams. The theory is that transdermal application rapidly delivers hormones into the small blood vessels of the dermis and speeds elimination.

Transdermal Patches

Commercially produced transdermal *patches* deliver hormones through the skin from a special controlled release gel within the patch. The patch releases the hormone at a fixed rate over several days. There are many commercial transdermal estradiol patches available on the Canadian market. Estraderm®, Estradot®, Estalis®, Oesclim®, and Climara® are all capable of delivering a measured amount of estradiol through the skin. Most require twice weekly dosing with the exception of Climara®, which is a once weekly patch. Studies show that transdermal estradiol patches give consistent serum and saliva levels over time. Some of the estradiol patches are used in combination with synthetic progestins. It is best to avoid patches with synthetic progestins because they differ from the body's own progesterone. Stick to the straight bio-identical estradiol patches!

Advantages: Delivery through skin is more similar to the body's own delivery of hormones than orally administered hormones. The main advantage of skin delivery is that it bypasses metabolism by the liver. Unlike oral forms, which are changed by the liver before they get to tissue, hormone creams tend to deliver the hormone key straight to the receptor lock. The biggest advantage of the transdermal *patch* is its consistent delivery of hormones over time. Transdermal delivery of estradiol has not been associated with the increase in triglycerides found with orally administered estradiol.

Disadvantages: Many people consider application of a cream or a gel to be an inconvenience. Patches are applied once or twice weekly, which is more convenient than daily or twice daily application of creams or gels, but some patients react to the adhesive on the patch, or find that the patch comes off unexpectedly. Transdermal patches are only available for estradiol and testosterone and the current testosterone patches are formulated in strengths appropriate for men, not women. Patches also lack the dosing flexibility of creams and gels since they come in fixed strengths. (Cutting the patch renders it ineffective.) Transdermal delivery of estradiol does not increase the *good* HDL cholesterol, as is the case with oral estrogens.

If the decision is made to deliver hormones through skin, the decision on whether to use transdermal patch, transdermal base or topical cream depends on the woman's preference and response to therapy. It is important to monitor response by regularly assessing symptoms and watching for potential problems (e.g. reaction to adhesive on transdermal patches). Unfortunately we do not have any data comparing the rate and effectiveness of hormone delivery between transdermal and topical bases.

We'll discuss some common bases used in bio-identical hormone replacement, and their specific properties. These are just a few representative examples; there are hundreds of different bases available.

Transdermal Bases
Transdermal bases contain chemical penetration enhancers that deliver the hormone deeper and more rapidly into the dermis than topical creams. Probably the most widely used enhancer is the liposome. Liposomes are small circular *droplets* that help carry drugs or hormones through the skin. The outside layer of the liposome is lipid loving (lipophilic) and therefore readily penetrates the layers of skin. Once through the skin, the liposome opens and delivers its contents to the capillaries (small blood vessels) for distribution to the tissues. Liposomes are not the only

enhancers of hormone delivery however. Other agents, such as esters, fatty acids, amides, alcohols, polyols, sulfoxides and even water, can assist in the delivery of hormones across skin cell membranes.

PLO gel is short for pluronic (or poloxamer F127) lecithin organogel. Properly prepared, PLO gel creates liposomes that effectively deliver hormone through the skin. There are a number of problems with the use of PLO gel to deliver hormones. The lecithin in PLO is derived from soy and some women may have an allergic reaction to soy. PLO gel is also very unappealing cosmetically and can leave a sticky film on the skin. These factors along with an alcohol odor and unpleasant texture led to the development of other transdermal creams.

Vanpen®, which is short for vanishing penetrate, is another common base for bio-identical hormone creams applied to the skin. It has a more pleasant texture and smell than the PLO gel, and still maintains enhanced transdermal properties. In addition to lecithin organogel, which forms liposomes, Vanpen® contains an ester and an amide. The ester assists liposome formation to ease the transport of hormone through skin. Urea, an amide, is also added to help moisturize the skin and increase its permeability to hormones. These enhancers work together to ensure that hormones successfully penetrate the skin layers and enter the capillaries of the dermis. Although rare, some people may react to ingredients found in Vanpen®. If an allergic reaction occurs, a hypoallergenic base called HRT Base® is available through pharmacies belonging to PCCA or Wiler-

PCCA (PCCA: Professional Compounding Centers of America; Wiler-PCCA: the Canadian sister organization– see Resources).

Topical Bases

Topical creams have no chemical penetration enhancers added. Because hormones are lipophilic (fat-loving), they tend to penetrate skin very well. The argument made for the use of topical bases is two-fold. First, they do not contain potential allergens in the form of chemical enhancers. Secondly, topical bases appear to deliver hormone only as far as the adipose (fat) cells in the dermis. The adipose cells store the fat-soluble hormone and tend to release it slowly as the need arises. Thus, topical hormones may deliver hormones in a more sustained release fashion that the transdermal bases. Note however, that there are no studies proving that topical bases actually result in a sustained release effect. Nevertheless, many compounding pharmacists and physicians who prescribe bio-identical hormones have reported that their patients experience more consistent symptom relief with topical hormone use compared to transdermal application.

Cosmetic HRT Base® is probably the most commonly used hormone cream base and is hypoallergenic, which means it is free of the most common allergy-provoking chemicals. It contains common cold cream ingredients, but with added natural vitamin E, plus vitamin C and A derivatives. This base is tolerated by virtually everyone. The water in Cosmetic HRT Base® helps to plump up the skin cells and

161

the resulting change in balance between lipids and water in the skin cell helps hormones to penetrate the skin.

TIPS FOR APPLYING HORMONE CREAMS

- Creams penetrate moist skin better than dry skin, so apply after a bath or shower (after towel drying)
- Creams penetrate *thin* skin better than *thick* skin, so apply to 'softer skin' like the inside of the arms. Skin that *blushes* is best.
- Applying to a large area is preferable to concentrating all the hormone in a small area.
- Don't apply hormone bases to abdominal skin, as this hormone may go directly to liver and form metabolites prior to delivery to tissue.
- Don't apply testosterone creams to the inner thighs as it might promote hair growth in this area.
- Applying progesterone cream to breast tissue may help reduce breast tissue density.
- Rotate through three or four different sites to avoid saturating the tissue in one area.
- Women should take a three to five-day break from progesterone cream each month to avoid developing a tolerance to its benefits. Taking a short break each month allows the progesterone to continue working.

Vaginal and Rectal Administration

Hormones delivered vaginally are well absorbed systemically (they are delivered to all body tissues) and provide detectable levels in both blood and saliva. Generally speaking however, hormones administered vaginally are used for their effects on vaginal tissue. That is, estrogens are given to help relieve vaginal dryness and progesterone is introduced vaginally to help maintain pregnancy. Estriol can also be used vaginally to help with incontinence. Creams, ointments, gels and suppositories are all used vaginally. Vaginal creams do not require chemical enhancers, because the lining of the vagina is a mucous membrane, which is considerably thinner and more permeable to hormones than exposed skin surfaces. Commercially available vaginal products include: Vagifem® vaginal estradiol tablet, and Crinone® 8% progesterone vaginal gel.

Hormones can also be administered rectally in the form of suspensions or as suppositories. Detectable levels of hormones are also achieved via this method, but most people consider this method messy and inconvenient.

***HRT Base*®** was discussed in detail under topical hormones. It is also used as a vaginal cream for the delivery of hormones. It contains no chemical enhancers and is hypoallergenic.

***Emollient Cream*®** is composed of about 50% water and is mixed with an anhydrous (water removed) ointment. An agent called an emulsifier is added to make sure that the ointment and the water mix properly and form a stable cream. Emollient Cream does not contain any chemical enhancers and is also hypoallergenic.

<u>Advantages:</u> Hormones are well absorbed via rectal or vaginal administration. Vaginal delivery of hormones is particularly useful when vaginal and urinary symptoms are predominant.

Disadvantages: This route of administration is can be inconvenient and messy.

Sublingual and Buccal

Sublingual delivery refers to the absorption of medication placed under the tongue. Buccal refers to placement of dosage forms between the gum and cheek. Sublingual and buccal dosage forms include lozenges (also called troches), drops, tablet triturates, and rapid dissolve tablets. With both sublingual and buccal forms, the rapid absorption of hormones may mean that doses need to be taken several times throughout the day in order to maintain therapeutic levels.

Sublingual Drops may be prepared using alcohol and glycerin solutions, oils or water-based suspensions. In order to keep the volume small, the hormone present in solution is very concentrated and therefore very bitter, in spite of flavouring agents.

Tablet Triturates are very small tablets designed to dissolve quickly when placed under the tongue or between the cheek and gums. The size of the tablet limits the amount of hormone that can be incorporated into it, and their manufacture is labour intensive.

Rapid Dissolve tablets are wafer-thin solid dosage forms also designed to dissolve quickly under the tongue or in the buccal cavity. They dissolve in as little as 10 seconds. They are easily flavoured to camouflage the bad taste, but are extremely fragile and difficult to handle.

Lozenges (Troches) take much longer to dissolve: up to 30 minutes depending on the type of base used. Gelatin bases dissolve more slowly than polyglycol bases, but the gelatin bases are more effective at concealing the bitter taste of the hormones.

Advantages: Rapid dissolve tablets and sublingual drops can avoid 'first pass' metabolism by the liver and the destruction of hormones by stomach acids.

Disadvantages: Sublingual and buccal forms are short acting, and they may need to be used up to three times daily to keep hormones at therapeutic levels. Because lozenges (troches) dissolve so slowly, patients end up swallowing a lot of hormone, which gets lost to stomach acid and liver metabolism. The tablet triturates don't hold a lot of hormone, and are expensive to make. With the exception of the Rapid Dissolve tablets, the sublingual and buccal forms cannot mask the unpleasant taste of hormones.

Injections and Implants

Therapeutic levels of hormones can be attained via injection. However, daily injections would be required to achieve consistent hormone levels over time. Consequently, long acting high dose injectables were developed, but these provide a decreasing dose of hormone over several weeks. Implants, like injections, require the use of high doses of hormones. In the case of implants, the hormone pellet is surgically placed under the skin, where it provides a slow release of hormones over a 3 to 6 month period.

Advantages: The main advantage of the injectable or implant forms is the convenience: dosing is infrequent (monthly, quarterly or semi-annually).

Disadvantages: The major disadvantage of injections and implants is that a large dose of hormone is given all at once. Patients experience very high hormone levels initially and then the hormone levels steadily decline until the next injection or implant, when there may be little or no hormone left. This method of administration in no way reflects the body's natural production of hormones and patients often experience side effects right after the injection or implant, and again when its effects wear off. The hormone pellet has to be surgically removed if there are any problems with tolerance or efficacy.

SUMMARY

Choosing a hormone delivery system is an important step in using bio-identical hormone replacement. It is generally best to use systems that deliver hormones in the way closest to natural hormone delivery. It is also important to use the right hormones, as determined by the symptom assessment and hormone test levels. Women who choose to use compounded hormones should deal with a pharmacy that is knowledgeable and experienced in compounding. Compounding pharmacies generally have specialized equipment to create these unique delivery systems. For example, some hormone powders are quite gritty and creams can also be gritty if they are not put through an ointment mill. This is another good reason to deal with a pharmacy that specializes in prescription compounding. Not all creams are created equal, particularly when it comes to delivering hormones!

RESOURCES

Recommended Reading

Lee, John *What Your Doctor May Not Tell You About Pre-Menopause*

Lee, John *What Your Doctor May Not Tell You About Menopause*

Lee, John and Zava, David *What Your Doctor May Not Tell You About Breast Cancer*

Northrup, Christiane *Women's Bodies, Women's Wisdom*

Northrup, Christiane *The Wisdom of Menopause*

Shippen, Eugene and Fryer, William *The Testosterone Syndrome: The Critical Factor for Energy, Health, & Sexuality – Reversing the Male Menopause.*

Wilson, James *Adrenal Fatigue: The 21St Century Syndrome*

Wright, Jonathan and Lenard, Lane *Maximize Your Vitality and Potency For Men Over 40*

Compounding Pharmacies
Wiler PCCA Canada

744 3rd Street
London, ON N5V 5J2
Ph: 519-455-0690

Website: www.pccarx.com

Find a list of member pharmacies under Links

International Academy of Compounding Pharmacists

Website: www.iacprx.org

Search by postal code or zip code to find a compounding pharmacist in your area.

Saliva Testing Laboratories

The following laboratories collect symptom information with each saliva test and give an interpretation of the results based on hormone levels and the symptom profile.

CANADA

Rocky Mountain Analytical

Unit A, 253147 Bearspaw Road NW
Calgary, Alberta T3L 2P5
Phone: 403-241-4513

Website: www.rmalab.com

UNITED STATES

ZRT Laboratory

1815 NW 169th Pl., Suite 505
Beaverton, Oregon 97006
Phone: 503-466-2445

Website: www.salivatest.com

REFERENCES

INTRODUCTION

Cundy T, Cornish J, Roberts H, et al. *Spinal bone density in women using depot medroxyprogesterone contraception.* Obstet Gynecol 1998;92:569-573.

Miyagawa K, Rosch J, Stanczyk F, Hermsmeyere K. *Medroxyprogesterone interferes with ovarian steroid protection against coronary vasospasm.* Nat Med 1997;3:324-327.

Williams J, Honore E, Washburn S, et al. *Effects of hormone replacement therapy on reactivity of atherosclerotic coronary arteries in cynomolgus monkeys.* J Am Coll Cardiol. 1994;224:1757-1761.

Writing Group for the Women's Health Initiative Investigators. *Risks and benefits of estrogen plus progestin in healthy postmenopausal women. Principal results from the Women's Health Initiative randomized controlled trial* JAMA 2002;288:321-333.

CHAPTER 1

Cushman M, Legault C, Barrett-Connor E, et al. *Effect of postmenopausal hormones on inflammation-sensitive proteins. The postmenopausal estrogen/progestin interventions (PEPI) study.* Circ 1999;100:717-722.

Hulley S, Grady D, Bush T, et al. *Randomized trial of estrogen plus progestin for secondary prevention of coronary heart disease in postmenopausal women. Heart and Estrogen/progestin Replacement Study (HERS) Research Group.* JAMA. 1998;280:605-613.

Lee W, Harder J, Yoshizumi M, et al. *Progesterone inhibits arterial smooth muscle cell proliferation.* Nat Med 1997;3:1005-1008.

Rosano G, Webb C, Chierchia S, et al. *Natural progesterone, but not medroxyprogesterone acetate, enhances the beneficial effect of estrogen on exercise-induced myocardial ischemia in postmenopausal women.* J Am Coll Cardiol 2000;36:2154-2159.

Writing Group for the Women's Health Initiative Investigators. *Risks and benefits of estrogen plus progestin in healthy postmenopausal women. Principal results from the Women's Health Initiative randomized controlled trial* JAMA 2002;288:321-333.

CHAPTER 2

Carlsen E. et al. *Evidence for decreasing quality of semen during past 50 years.* BMJ. 1992;305:609-613.

Head KA. *Estriol: safety and efficacy.* Altern Med Rev. 1998;3:101-113.

Herman-Giddens ME et al. *Secondary sexual characteristics and menses in young girls seen in office practice: a study from the Pediatric Research in Office Settings network.* Pediatrics 1997;99:505-512.

Skakkebaek N.E. et al. *Should We Watch What We Eat and Drink? Report on the International Workshop on Hormones and Endocrine Disrupters in Food and Water: Possible Impact on Human Health, Copenhagen, Denmark, 27-30 May 2000.*Trends Endocrinol Metab 2000;11:291-293.

Taylor M. *Unconventional estrogens: Estriol, Biest and Triest.* Clin Obstet Gynecol 2001;44:864-879.

CHAPTER 3

Arlt W, Callies F, van Vlijmen J, Koehler I, et al. *Dehydroepiandrosterone replacement in women with adrenal insufficiency.* N Engl J Med 1999 Sep 30;341(14):1013-1020.

Davis S, McCloud P, Strauss B, Burger H. *Testosterone enhances estradiol's effects on postmenopausal bone density and sexuality.* Maturitas 1995 Apr;21(3):227-236.

Miller B, De Souza M, Slade K, Luciano A. *Sublingual administration of micronized estradiol and progesterone, with and without micronized testosterone: effect on biochemical markers of bone metabolism and bone mineral density.* Menopause 2000 Sep-Oct;7(5):318-326.

Scott L, Salahuddin F, Cooney J, et al. *Differences in adrenal steroid profile in chronic fatigue syndrome, in depression and in health.* J Affect Disord 1999;54:129-137.

Shifren J, Braunstein G, Simon J, et al. *Transdermal testosterone treatment in women with impaired sexual function after oophorectomy.* N Engl J Med 2000 Sep 7;343(10):682-688.

Suzuki M, Kanazawa A, Hasegawa M, et al. *A close association between insulin resistance and dehydroepiandrosterone sulfate in subjects with essential hypertension.* Endocr J 1999;46:521-528.

Tagawa N, Tamanaka J, Fujinami A, et al. *Serum dehydroepiandrosterone, dheydroepiandrosterone sulphate, and pregnenolone sulfate concentrations in patients with hyperthyroidism and hypothyroidism.* Clin Chem 2000;46:523-528.

CHAPTER 4

Arrenbrecht S, Boermans A. *Effects of transdermal estradiol delivered by a matrix patch on bone density in hysterectomized, postmenopausal women: a 2 –year placebo-controlled trial.* Osteoporos Int 2002;13:176-183.

Cavalieri E, Rogan E, Chakravarti D. *Initiation of cancer and other diseases by catechol ortho-quinones: a unifying mechanism.* Cell Mol Life Sci 2002;59:665-681.

Chang K, Lee T, Linares-Cruz G. *Influences of percutaneous administration of estradiol and progesterone on human breast epithelial cell cycle in vivo.* Fertil Steril 1995;63.785-791.

Cushman M, Legault C, Barrett-Connor E, et al. *Effect of postmenopausal hormones on inflammation-sensitive proteins. The postmenopausal estrogen/progestin interventions (PEPI) study.* Circ 1999;100:717-722.

Gavin N, Thorp J, Ohsfeldt R. *Determinants of hormone replacement therapy duration among postmenopausal women with intact uteri.* Menopause. 2001;8:377-383.

Granberg S, Eurenius K, Lindgren R, Wilhelmsson L. *The effects of oral estriolon the endometrium in postmenopausal women.* Maturitas 2002;42:149-156.

Head KA. *Estriol: safety and efficacy.* Altern Med Rev. 1998;3:101-113.

Honisett S, Pang B, Stojanovska L, et al. *Progesterone does not influence vascular function in postmenopausal women.* J Hypertens 2003;21:1145-1149.)

Iosif CS. *Effects of protracted estriol administration on the lower genito urinary tracts of postmenopausal women.* Arch Gynecol Obstet 1992;251(3):115-20

Landes J, Leonetti H, Anasti J. *Topical Progesterone Cream: An Alternative Progestin in Hormone Replacement Therapy.* Abstract of Third Prize Paper: Monday Papers - Obstetrics & Gynecology April 2003: p 65.

Lee W, Harder J, Yoshizumi M, et al. *Progesterone inhibits arterial smooth muscle cell proliferation.* Nat Med 1997;3:1005-1008.

Leonetti H, Longo S, Anasti J. *Transdermal progesterone cream for vasomotor symptoms and postmenopausal bone loss.* Obstet Gynecol 1999;94:225-228.

Leonetti H, Wilson J, Anasti J. *Topical progesterone cream has an antiproliferative effect on estrogen-stimulated endometrium.* Fertil Steril 2003;79:221-222.

Lundstrom E, Wilczek B, von Palffy Z, et al. *Mammographic breast density during hormone replacement therapy: effects of continuous combination, unopposed transdermal and low-potency estrogen regimens.* Climacteric. 2001;4:42-48.

Medina D. *Breast cancer: the protective effect of pregnancy.* Clin Cancer Res. 2004 Jan 1;10(1 Pt 2):380S-4S.

173

Montplaisir J, Lorrain J, Denesle R, Petit D. *Sleep in menopause: differential effects of two forms of hormone replacement therapy.* Menopause: J N Am Meno Soc 2001;8:10-16.

Reed M, Purohit A. *Breast cancer and the role of cytokines in regulating estrogen synthesis: an emerging hypothesis.* Endocr Rev 1997;18:701-715.

Rosano G, Webb C, Chierchia S, et al. *Natural progesterone, but not medroxyprogesterone acetate, enhances the beneficial effect of estrogen on exercise-induced myocardial ischemia in postmenopausal women.* J Am Coll Cardiol 2000;36:2154-2159.

Seeger H, Wallwiener D, Mueck AO. *Effect of medroxyprogesterone acetate and norethisterone on serum-stimulated and estradiol-inhibited proliferation of human coronary artery smooth muscle cells.* Menopause 2001;8:5-9.

Somers, S. *The Sexy Years.* Crown Publishers, New York, NY. 2004

Takahashi K, Okada M, Ozaki T, et al. *Safety and efficacy of oestriol for symptoms of natural or surgically induced menopause.* Hum Reprod 2000;15:1028-1036.

Taylor M. *Unconventional estrogens: Estriol, Biest and Triest.* Clin Obstet Gynecol 2001;44:864-879.

Ursin G. et al. *Reproductive factors and risk of breast carcinoma in a study of white and African-American women.* Cancer. 2004 Jul 15;101(2):353-62.

Utsumi T, Yoshimura N, Takeuchi S, et al. *Elevated steroid sulphatase expression in breast cancers.* J Steroid Biochem Mol Biol 2000;73:141-145.

Waddell B, O'Leary P. *Distribution and metabolism of topically applied progesterone in a rat model.* J Steroid Biochem Mol Biol 2002;80:449-455.

Writing Group for the Women's Health Initiative Investigators. *Risks and benefits of estrogen plus progestin in healthy postmenopausal women. Principal results from the Women's Health Initiative randomized controlled trial* JAMA 2002;288:321-333.

CHAPTER 5

Leiblum S, Bachmann G, Kemmann Eet al. *Vaginal atrophy in the postmenopausal woman. The importance of sexual activity and hormones.* JAMA 1983;249:2195-2198.

Lemon H. *Pathophysiologic considerations in the treatment of menopausal patients with oestrogens; the role of oestriol in the prevention of mammary carcinoma.* Acta Endocrinol Suppl (Copenh)1980;233:17-27.

Melamed M, Castano E, Notides A, et al. *Molecular and kinetic basis for the mixed agonist/antagonist activity of estriol.* Mol Endocrinol. 1997;11:1868-1878.

Mohr P, Wang D, Gregory W, et al. *Serum progesterone and prognosis in operable breast cancer.* Br J Cancer 1996;73:1552-1555.

Ottoson U, Carlstrom K, Damber J, von Schoultz B. *Serum levels of progesterone and some of its metabolites including deoxycorticosterone after oral and parenteral administration.* Br J Obstet Gynaecol 1984;91:1111-1119.

Pol-Kantola P. *When does estrogen replacement therapy improve sleep quality?* Am J Obstet Gynecol 1998 May;178(5):1002-9

Schwingl PJ. *Risk factors for menopausal hot flashes.* Obstet Gynecol 1994 Jul;84(1):29-34

CHAPTER 9

Gambineri A. et al *Testosterone levels in obese male patients with obstructive sleep apnea syndrome: relation to oxygen desaturation, body weight, fat distribution and the metabolic parameters.*
J Endocrinol Invest. 2003 Jun;26(6):493-8.

Giordano S et al. *Breast cancer in men.* Ann Int Med 2002; 137 (8): 678-687

Malkin C, Pugh P, Morris P, et al. *Testosterone replacement in hypogonadal men with angina improves ischaemic threshold and quality of life.* Heart 2004;90:871-876.

Massengill JC. *Pretreatment testosterone level predicts pathological stage in patients with localized prostate cancer treated with radical prostatectomy.* J Urol 2003May;169(5):1670-5

Morales A. *The Andropause: Bare Facts for Urologists.* BJU Int 2003 Mar;91(4)31:311-313

Morales A. Tenover JL. *Androgen deficiency in the aging male: when, who, and how to investigate and treat.* Urol Clin North Am 2002 Nov;29(4):975-82

Morgan C, Wang S, Mason J et al. *Hormone profiles in humans experiencing military survival training.* Biol Psychiatry 2000;47:891-901

Morgentaler A. Bruning CO. *Occult prostate cancer in men with low serum testosterone levels.* JAMA 1996Dec 18;276(23):1904-6.

Perry P. *Bioavailable Tesosterone as a Correlate of Cognition, Psychological Status, Quality of Life, and Sexual Function in Aging Males: Implications for Testosterone Replacement Therapy.* Ann Clin Psych 2001;13(2):75-80

Plymate SR et al. *Circadian variation in testosterone, sex hormone-binding globulin, and calculated non-sex hormone-binding globulin bound testosterone in healthy young and elderly men.* J Andrology. 1989 Sep-Oct;10(5):366-71

Prehn R. *On the Prevention and Therapy of Prostate Cancer by Androgen Administration.* Cancer Research 1999 Sept 1;59:4161-4164

Tremblay R, Morales A. *Canadian practice recommendations for screening, monitoring and treating men affected by andropause or partial androgen deficiency.* The Aging Male 1998;1:213-218.

Vermeulen A. *Diagnosis of partial androgen deficiency in the aging male.* Ann Endocrinol (Pari). 2003 Apr;64(2):109-14

INDEX